T0323497

The Private Life of the Genome

This innovative and engaging book argues that because our genetic information is directly linked to the genetic information of others, it is impossible to assert a "right to privacy" in the same way that we can in other areas of life.

This position throws up questions around access to sensitive data. It suggests that we may have to abandon certain intuitions about who may access our genetic information; and it raises concerns about discrimination against people with certain genetic characteristics. But the author asserts that regulating access to genetic information requires a more nuanced perspective that does not rely on the familiar language of rights. The book proposes new ways in which we may think about who has access to what genetic information, and on what basis they do so.

Conceptually challenging, the book will prove engaging reading for scholars and students interested in the area of bioethics and medical law, as well as policy makers working with these pressing issues.

Iain Brassington is a Senior Lecturer at the Centre for Social Ethics and Policy in the Department of Law at the University of Manchester, UK.

The Private Life of the Genome

Genetic Information and the Right to Privacy

Iain Brassington

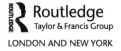
Routledge
Taylor & Francis Group

LONDON AND NEW YORK

First published 2023
by Routledge
4 Park Square, Milton Park, Abingdon, Oxon OX14 4RN

and by Routledge
605 Third Avenue, New York, NY 10158

Routledge is an imprint of the Taylor & Francis Group, an informa business

© 2023 Iain Brassington

British Library Cataloguing-in-Publication Data
A catalogue record for this book is available from the British Library

ISBN: 978-1-032-32044-1 (hbk)
ISBN: 978-1-032-32043-4 (pbk)
ISBN: 978-1-003-31251-2 (ebk)

DOI: 10.4324/9781003312512

Typeset in Goudy
by MPS Limited, Dehradun

Contents

Acknowledgements

The preparation of this book has been glacially slow, the blame for which lies mainly with me, partly with the Courts: having realised that I could not get the manuscript ready for publication before ABC was heard a second time I felt I had to wait for that case to be decided in order not to be caught out by it, and partly with SARS-cov-2, which has snared up everything, and provided an alibi for any number of missed deadlines around the world since 2020. Nevertheless, that it was produced even as quickly as it was is attributable to the help and support of a number of people. In the first place, I must thank my father, Phillip Brassington, for having kept prodding me. I owe a huge debt of thanks, too, to my colleagues at Manchester – in particular to Søren Holm, Simona Giordano, Catherine Stanton, Jonathan Lewis, Bruce Wardhaugh, Jean d'Aspremont, and Yenkong Hodu, who variously read drafts and fragments, and provided suggestions, encouragement, and general chivvying-on, and to Emma Hilton, who provided useful nudges about how genetics works in practice. Thanks also to Emily Postan and Tuija Takala, who provided very valuable external feedback. I think I ought also to mention Graham Smeaton, whose suggested title for the book – "Unzipped Genes" – I have used as a header for the introduction. Whether this is an acknowledgement or an attempt to share the blame, I am not sure.

Chapter 3 revisits and reworks my 2011 paper "Is There a Duty to Remain in Ignorance?" (*Theoretical Medicine and Bioethics* 32[2]: 101–115); chapter 6 revisits my 2014 paper "Genetic Information: Making a Just World Strange" (*Theoretical Medicine and Bioethics* 35[3]: 231–246).

Introduction: Unzipped Genes

Genetic information is quick, easy, and cheap to obtain. America's National Human Genome Research Institute publishes data every year on the costs of sequencing a Megabase of DNA and a genome the size of the human genome. In September 2001, a Megabase cost a shade over $5292 to sequence. By August 2021, sequencing one Megabase would cost just over half a cent, and a whole human genome a princely $562.[1] Meanwhile, 23andMe is one of a number of companies to offer direct-to-consumer (DtC) genetic testing on a commercial basis. Customers can post a saliva sample to the company, and in six to eight weeks receive a report on their ancestry and health-related genetic markers. UK customers will pay £149 for the health and ancestry service[2]; Americans pay $199.[3] The advances in genetic technology made over the last couple of decades have been astonishing; the increased access that that gives us to genetic information equally so.

The way in which we think about how to handle that information has not kept up.

At least, that is the concern that motivates my argument in this book. We care about privacy, and we worry that sensitive information about us will be available to other people; we like to think that we have rights to privacy in respect of this information. But information about our genes is not straightforwardly and only about us, and this makes many claims about rights to privacy (at least in this context) hard to sustain. I want to make the case that there is no *ab initio* moral right to genetic privacy; any "right" we have in this respect is the product of, rather than a *datum* in, moral discussion: it is not a consideration that trumps or is even to be weighed against other considerations. Questions about how or whether we ought to protect rights to privacy therefore miss the important issue. And though the language of rights does have a certain utility when talking about who may access what information and under what circumstances, I shall argue that it does so only as a shorthand for other concerns: when we say that Alice has a right to privacy in respect of some aspect of her genetic information, this is a way of saying that the balance of moral considerations is that other people are not entitled to access that information.

The position at which I shall arrive is not that it is wrong to access genetic information about a person when and because they have a right to privacy in

DOI: 10.4324/9781003312512-1

respect of it, but that they have a right to privacy in respect of genetic information when and because others accessing it would be (all things considered) wrong. The things to be considered include the nature of the information, the reason why it is to be accessed, who will learn what, and so on. When tackling questions about who has or ought to have what kind of control over and access to genetic information, we ought to think about agents as having interests that have weight, and reasons that have importance, *in a context*. Crucially, part of that context will involve a network of other persons with their own potentially competing and overlapping interests – and some of those other persons will be relatives with whom agents share their genes in a reasonably predictable way. Working out right and wrong will depend on measuring all these interests against each other and reconciling any competition between them in the best way possible, noting that how we should understand "best" may itself be open to debate.

A consequence of this claim is that the "rights" in play will change from person to person, from context to context, and depending on the kind of information and the reason why it may be shared. A further consequence will be that, if we are inclined to put guidelines about the use and protection of genetic information into formal regulatory instruments or statutes, we ought to be prepared for those guidelines to have quite a bit of room for interpretation and the application of context-appropriate judgement; for them not to have such room would mean that they would come apart from our moral intuitions at least reasonably often, with the attendant damage that that would do for their being taken seriously.

At the core of my claim is an observation about the way that we currently tend to think about genetic information. Many of the ethical tools brought to bear on questions of access to genetic information are borrowed from other areas within biomedical ethics; but these tools are often inappropriate or, at least, not used well.

Importantly, most biomedical information is (to coin a phrase) "confined". By this, I mean that it tells us nothing by its nature about anyone else. For example, if Alice knows that Benny has had his appendix out, she will not learn anything about whether his relatives Jenny, Kenny, Lenny, or Penny have also had theirs removed. Unsurprisingly, because most biomedical information is confined, most of the tools we have for thinking about how to handle it assume confinement. But this stores up problems in respect of unconfined information – information that by its nature *can* tell us something about others without their having to provide any supplementary information of their own – that the familiar tools are ill-fitted to solve; and genetic information is unconfined. Moreover, not only are the familiar ethical tools potentially unreliable when it comes to handling genetic information: their use may even generate new problems – a point I shall explore in chapter 3.

It's worth taking a moment to distinguish between genetic *data* and genetic *information*. The word "information" in everyday use could mean the raw data about a person's genome, say as a printout of As, Cs, Gs, and Ts; or it could mean what we get when those data are processed, enabling us to talk about a person's carrying a gene associated with this or that characteristic. This slight ambiguity can be resolved by reserving the word "data" for unprocessed material; "information" is what data become once they are processed. Generally, it is information that will concern me, because information is the more ready-to-hand and the source of most everyday concerns. It's what the bare data *mean* in practice – how they are and can be refined into information and put to use, and the impact of that use on actual lives – that matters.

The argument I shall make will draw on a handful of real-life legal cases for illustrative purposes, but it is for the most part an exercise in moral philosophy. Equally, though what I have to say may well have implications in healthcare practice and for those whose work is in or touches upon healthcare practice, I shall have little to say about professional guidelines except as a way to get discussion going in the early stages of the book, and to take a quick look at what some of the implications of the argument may be in its final pages.

Naturally, there are things I shall not address; some readers will find these omissions to be a source of criticism. For example, I have little to say about the use of genetic information and privacy more generally in "big data" projects. This is because the concerns raised there are for the most part either not specific to genetic information, or bigger than the problems of genetic information. For consideration of privacy in this context, I would point readers in the direction of the 2019 special edition of the *Asian Bioethics Review* devoted to the SHAPES working group on big data in health and research, and, of course, of Shoshana Zuboff's magisterial book on "surveillance capitalism".[4]

And other readers will be dissatisfied with the moral theoretical positions I have adopted. They will want to insist that there *is* something to a right (or a right to genetic privacy) that is more substantial than "whatever it is that we are left with when we bash the relevant claims and interests together" – which is more or less the position I have adopted. And to this, I can do little but to hold up my hands: my account of rights (or this right, at least) is where the argument has led me, but there is more theoretical work to be done. This book is already plenty long enough; filling in the theoretical gaps is an important task, but it will have to wait its turn. That said, whatever we think there is to be said or would want to say about what a right is, how we come to possess a right, the relationship between a right and human dignity, and so on, there will remain the problem of what to do when two agents have interests, which we may want to call rights, that are equal and opposite. My positions here depart from the observation that genetic information may put us in the position of having to decide what to do then.

Notes

1 Data available to download via https://www.genome.gov/about-genomics/fact-sheets/DNA-Sequencing-Costs-Data; last checked 24.v.22.
2 https://www.23andme.com/en-gb/?evr=epv; checked 24.v.22.
3 https://www.23andme.com/?evr=epv; checked 24.v.22.
4 Zuboff, S, *The Age of Surveillance Capitalism* (London: Profile, 2019).

Part I

Presumptions and Foundations

1   Genes and Information-Sharing

We tend to think that privacy is a good – as Anita Allen puts it, "a basic and foundational human good meriting moral and legal protection"[1]: something to which moral rights attach and to which legal rights should attach. A great deal of ink has been spilled looking at ways to ensure that privacy is protected; that it is something that *ought* to be protected is more or less a given. Violations of privacy are threats: the word "violation" itself connotes as much. The main thrust of this book is to articulate problems with the idea of a thoroughgoing right to privacy in respect of genetic information. An important part of making this case, and one that will occupy a good deal of this chapter, is to argue that there is a "standard model" of bioethics that delineates the conventional ways to think about practical problems, including those arising in respect of handling potentially sensitive information. I shall suggest that the standard model is wanting when it comes to genetic information, because it struggles to account for the fact that genetic information displays a characteristic that I shall call "unconfinement". I shall explain more a little later what I mean by "unconfined" information; but I shall start to set out the argument in a familiar place.

i. Two Cases

Perhaps the most famous legal case to deal with the control of medically sensitive information is that of *Tarasoff*.[2] The bare facts of this case are that a patient, Prosenjit Poddar, had told his therapist of his intentions to kill Tatiana Tarasoff. That information was passed to police authorities, but not to Tarasoff herself, or to her family. Poddar was detained briefly, but released when he was assessed not to be a threat; he killed Tarasoff a short time later. Her family sued the therapist and various others, drawing on the claim that they had had a duty to share the information they had about Poddar more widely.[3] The core of the matter considered can be captured as a few questions. First, should Poddar have been at liberty to begin with? Second, is it permissible for therapists to disclose the fact that a patient has threatened a third party, for the sake of protecting that third party? Third, if so, what information may be shared? Fourth, to whom?

DOI: 10.4324/9781003312512-3

In considering these questions, the Court had to weigh in the balance the pros and cons of allowing Poddar his liberty, and of disclosing information. On the liberty front, the judgment maintained that the possibility of future violence from an agent cannot be taken as a reason to deprive that agent of his liberty, since that principle would imperil the freedom of all. But in finding for the plaintiffs, Justice Torbriner noted that there were alternatives to detention available, and in doing so referred to deprivation of liberty as "drastic".[4] He also reasoned that while issuing a warning that proved unnecessary might be damaging, the risk was a reasonable one to take if a life were at stake.[5] In his dissenting opinion, Justice Clark also gave voice to a concern about patients being committed unnecessarily; but he was also worried that to insist on a duty to warn could actually *increase* rates of unnecessary commitment, since it might incline therapists to commit a patient who would not otherwise have been committed in order to avoid having to make a prediction about the threat that that patient posed, and opening themselves up to liability claims in the event of making a wrong call.[6] This would undermine the principle of liberty that the whole bench sought to uphold. He also suggested that imposing a duty to warn might disincline patients from seeking treatment, and that, since there would likely be some patients who would be a threat without treatment but who would not present (as much of) a threat with it, such a disinclination might actually mean that the danger posed to the public increased.[7]

As we can see, the interests of psychiatric patients in feeling that they could trust their therapist, and the associated therapeutic reason to maintain privilege, were in competition with the interests of the public to protection. In the end, the decision taken was that information should have been shared more widely, Justice Torbriner noting in the majority argument that

> when a therapist determines, or pursuant to the standards of his profession should determine, that his patient presents a serious danger of violence to another, he incurs an obligation to use reasonable care to protect the intended victim against such danger.[8]

"More widely" does not imply "particularly widely". One might think that any moral entitlement to be warned was held by Tarasoff herself, but nobody else; conceivably, one might think that it was held by the police but not by Tarasoff. Either way, as the majority opinion continued,

> [w]e recognize the public interest in supporting effective treatment of mental illness and in protecting the rights of patients to privacy. [...] Against this interest, however, we must weigh the public interest in safety from violent assault. [...]
>
> We conclude that the public policy favoring protection of the confidential character of patient-psychotherapist communications must

yield to the extent to which disclosure is essential to avert danger to others. The protective privilege ends where the public peril begins.[9]

While not all the judges hearing the case agreed that information should have been shared, there was no clear rejection of the terms on which the decision had been made; the minority opinion centred largely on the interpretation and application of statute.

The framework around which the judgment was reached was one in which the claims of each party were considered and balanced against each other, and against the desirability of sharing information, both in this case and as a matter of principle. As we see from the quotation above, it was held in this case that "[t]he protective privilege ends where the public peril begins".[10] But an important aspect of the judgment was its acceptance that, while it may have been permissible or even required to breach privilege in this case, such a move would have been exceptional: there is a principle of maintaining privilege that *on this occasion* must give way. To say that a principle must give way is to accept that there is a principle all the same. To borrow reasoning from Cicero, if there is an exception that makes a course of action permissible, that course of action would by implication not be permissible absent the exception.[11]

To summarise: though this case actually hinged on matters of the interpretation of statute and precedent, we can see in the language of the judgment many appeals to certain moral precepts, the best interests of the patient, the best interests of society at large, and the importance of privacy and of liberty being important among them. And while it was accepted that Poddar should not have been detained, it was also held that it would have been appropriate to share certain information to a certain limited number of people. He did have arguable claims not to have sensitive information broadcast, but they were not the only consideration.

The *Tarasoff* ruling was cited with approval in a more recent case before the English Courts that speaks to concerns about how to handle genetic information: *ABC v St George's Healthcare NHS Trust.* This case concerned a suit brought against St George's by a woman referred to as ABC, daughter of a man, XX, who was serving a sentence for the manslaughter of her mother. XX had been diagnosed with Huntington's Disease in November 2009, and this information had not been passed on. Due to an accidental disclosure, ABC learned of the diagnosis a little under a year later, in August 2010 – but not before having given birth to a child in April of that year. Huntington's being an autosomal dominant condition, there was a 50% chance that ABC had inherited it, and – if she had – a 50% chance that she would pass it on to her child. Had she known of the risk, she claimed, she would have had herself tested; and had she tested positive for the gene, she would have terminated the pregnancy.[12] ABC's contention was that knowledge of her father's condition was germane to her continuation of the pregnancy, that she therefore had a right to have been told about it before the accidental disclosure, and that not having been told about it therefore represented a wrong. XX, for his part, had decided against sharing at least in part because he feared that ABC would terminate her pregnancy, and he did not want her to do that.

The judgment at the first instance went against ABC's having had the right to be told about XX's diagnosis. One of the considerations important in Mr Justice Nicol's reasoning was the confidential nature of the information in question. ABC, he allowed, did have an interest in having been told about her father's diagnosis –

> there is plainly a balance to be stuck between the value to the Claimant of knowing that her father had this genetic condition on the one hand and her father's right to have the confidentiality of his medical information preserved[13]

but he found that on this occasion, it was the father's interest that prevailed, not least because he was unpersuaded that the Trust had a duty of care towards the daughter. On appeal, the daughter's arguments were found by the bench to be more compelling than Nicol J had found them, and the case was remitted for trial.

The case was heard for the second time in 2020, and in her opinion Mrs Justice Yip reasserted the "strong public interest in respecting medical confidentiality which extends beyond the privacy of the individual patient",[14] but noted also that Article 8 rights to respect for private and family life pull in two directions, generating both a legal right to medical confidentiality that would prevent disclosure to XX's daughter, and a right to have information about one's own health that lent weight to the daughter's claim to access.[15] Ultimately finding against ABC, Yip J noted that though she *was* owed a duty of care by the second defendant, South West London and St George's Mental Health NHS Trust, this extended as far as *considering* her interest in knowing about her father's genetic test result, and balancing that against the public interest in keeping controls on information flow. "The decision not to disclose," she found, "was supported by a responsible body of medical opinion and was a matter of judgment open to the second defendant after balancing the competing interests".[16] In both hearings, a great deal of weight was placed on the professional ethical guidance in helping reach a decision, and on a construal of the *ethos* of the profession. Yip J made an appeal to the standards set out by a responsible body of medical opinion; both she and Nicol J had quoted at length from the report by the Royal College of Physicians, Royal College of Pathologists and British Society for Human Genetics' Joint Commission on Medical Genetics published in 2006, *Consent and Confidentiality in Genetic Practice*.[17] This report, which set the standard for practice at the time of the breach, granted that maintaining confidentiality in situations in which information about one person might affect another would be the default, but admitted that disclosure might be permissible under certain circumstances; it stipulated, though, that the risk of harm from non-disclosure must outweigh the distress caused by disclosure to the patient.[18] (The 2011 iteration of the report came to substantially the same conclusion, though framed it in terms of balancing the public interest in disclosure with the public interest in maintaining confidentiality[19]; neither did the 2019 iteration depart from this, saying that

> [i]n certain circumstances it may be justified to break confidence where the avoidance of harm by the disclosure outweighs the patient's claim to confidentiality. This principle has been reiterated in a recent legal case in which the Court of Appeal stated that it may have been potentially justifiable for a health professional to breach the confidentiality of their patient in order to benefit others.[20]

(It is perhaps worth noting that who those others are is not elaborated; neither is any detail given about the scale on which relative interests are to be weighed.)

The JCMG reports draw from the guidance offered by the statutory regulator, the General Medical Council. The GMC's guidance from the time of the earliest of the JCMG's reports stated that

> [p]ersonal information may be disclosed in the public interest, without patients' consent, and in exceptional cases where patients have withheld consent, if the benefits to an individual or to society of the disclosure outweigh both the public and the patient's interest in keeping the information confidential. You must weigh the harms that are likely to arise from non-disclosure of information against the possible harm, both to the patient and to the overall trust between doctors and patients, arising from the release of that information.[21]

The most recent iteration of the guidance states, similarly, that

> [i]n exceptional circumstances, there may be an overriding public interest in disclosing personal information without consent for important health and social care purposes if there is no reasonably practicable alternative to using personal information and it is not practicable to seek consent. The benefits to society arising from the disclosure must outweigh the patient's and public interest in keeping the information confidential

although it adds that "the circumstances in which the public interest would justify such disclosures are uncertain".[22] One may wonder whether a healthcare professional would find in such advice a clear instruction about what to do: it describes the contours of the problem, noting that there is a balance to be struck between competing interests and entitlements; but on *how* to strike that balance, there is much less. Neither – in defence of the GMC – is it obvious what *could* be said, since it is likely that cases will be different and that this difference will militate against there being a clear and easy-to-articulate rubric. That point will prove important in the final chapter of this book.

The important point for my purposes is that ABC – like *Tarasoff* – had to do with who was entitled to what kind of access to what information. Of course, there are differences between *Tarasoff* and ABC. Not the least of them is that in the earlier case, the plaintiffs' claim that they should have been informed was upheld, and in the latter, the plaintiff's claim that she should have been told (or told sooner, and deliberately) was rejected. But there are important similarities, too. The judicial reasoning in both draws on questions of trust, confidentiality, the existence and nature of a duty to protect, and so on. In essence, it is an account of who owes what to whom. And in both, although a case might be made for sharing medically sensitive information about a person without their permission, the case *does* have to be made. Absent that case's being made, the person to whom information refers most proximately – its primary referent – has authority over it. Even if ABC had been decided differently, and it had been held that the information about XX's diagnosis should have been shared with ABC, that is not the same as its having been decided that he did not have all-else-being-equal authority over it. An exception to the rule would have been identified, but – as I have posited – an exception to a rule shows only that there is a rule. A question that does linger, though, has to do with exactly who is the referent of a given piece of genetic information, a matter that will clearly be important if we think that the referent has authority over who gets access and under what circumstances.

A quick *précis* of two cases is, of course, fairly small beer in the grand scheme of things. Nevertheless, it does enable me to move to the next part of setting out my stall, which is that these cases reflect a certain prevalent way of approaching bioethical questions. Having outlined some features of this "standard model", I shall then be able to take my first steps to showing how and why it breaks down in respect of genetic information.

ii. Features of a "Standard Model" of Bioethics

There is across bioethics – at least, anglophone bioethics – a "standard" way of thinking about not only how to answer practical questions, but also about how to frame them in the first place. Loosely, this model places the individual as the centre of moral concern; though there are some bioethicists with a more communitarian outlook who demur from the model, it is safe to say that we assume that even when moral agents have duties, they are nevertheless morally separable from those around them. Concepts like autonomy (and respect for autonomy) play their role within the standard model: they set the terms of how we decide what one person may or may not do to another, and they grant to the individual a protection against physical, psychological, and moral intrusion; they ensure the agent's "integrity". Even if we think that someone ought to do something, we also presume that those duties are things that attach to agents who can be thought of as moral isolates. Thus I might have duties, but they are *my* duties, and you cannot generally force me to discharge them without violating my integrity. Kant is the most obvious parent of this sort of model of moral thinking,[23] but Millian thought behaves in the same sort of way: as *On Liberty* has it, over himself the individual is sovereign.[24]

Beauchamp and Childress's *Principles of Biomedical Ethics* is, for better or worse, at the centre of the standard model. The "principlist" account derived from it is firmly rooted in, and is an expression of, the standard model. The project of the *Principles* is to codify the terms of bioethical debate by synthesising what had come before, and by naming four principles – respect for autonomy, beneficence, non-maleficence, and justice – around which the ethical edifice is built. Beauchamp and Childress's claim is that these principles can be deduced from what they call a "common morality" – a set of precepts that they hold would be found in any recognisable moral system – and that (particularly when supplemented with processes of reflective equilibrium) they can generate more specific sets of moral rules.[25] Some earlier editions of the *Principles* attempted to arrange the principles into a table, and to correlate them with a range of rules, virtues, and ideals. The table offered in the sixth edition[26] does not appear in the seventh; but the difference between obligation and supererogation is put into another table in the later version.[27] Beauchamp and Childress can be seen as trying to take the "particles" of recognisable moral theories, and arrange them in a way that is reminiscent of the way that physicists arrange bosons, leptons, and quarks into a standard model of subatomic reality. Officially, they offer no hierarchy of their principles, taking it as enough to offer them as an explanation for the way that bioethical discussion does and should play out. Unofficially, and in keeping with liberal axioms, respect for autonomy is often taken to be the *sine qua non* of decent behaviour, and showing that some proposed course of action is in tension with the principle, let alone antagonistic to it, is taken as evidence against doing it. Raanan Gillon gives his explicit approval to the proposition that bioethics needs the four principles, but that respect for autonomy should be regarded as *primus inter pares*.[28] Whatever the normative force of this position, as an expression of the way the model works in the real world, it is probably right: beneficence and non-maleficence are understood as expressions of what autonomous agents may and may not do to each other, and justice regulates the interactions of autonomous (and therefore morally equal) agents.

When it comes to questions about who has control over access to information, under what conditions, and with what limits, a cursory glance at the literature indicates that the standard model is often applied. Information such as that contained in things like medical records "belongs" to its primary referent, who usually has the ultimate say in who has access to it. Departures from that default position threaten the integrity of individuals, and are therefore undesirable; deliberately to infringe on that integrity is a wrong except when not doing so will itself imperil another's integrity; and when an infringement is unwitting or unavoidable, there is a moral imperative to mitigate and minimise it – to keep as much of the genie in the bottle as possible. Often this approach is articulated in terms of rights: hence persons have rights, related to the principle of respect for autonomy, to privacy and confidentiality; these rights can be brought to moral debate to prevent others getting access to information, and can be deployed as reasons to maximise the referent's control.

The standard model can accommodate exceptions to the maintenance of privacy and confidentiality when there is deemed to be a good moral reason to share information. What counts as a good moral reason would be a matter for further debate; but protecting the immediate welfare of a third party may well be the sort of thing that counts. As indicated a moment ago, exceptions to primary referents' control over information would apply primarily when another agent's integrity is put at risk, and to the extent necessary to restore and guarantee that integrity as far as possible. Of course, not all information-sharing is a threat to the integrity of the referent: telling a new recruit in an office how to identify colleagues is perfectly permissible, even though it is technically sharing information about them. Finally, it is likely to be the case that even sensitive information can be shared without explicit permission in some circumstances: for example, members of a medical team have good reason to share medical information about me to the extent that it is relevant to the treatment they are providing, and may generally do so without my having to approve it. Nevertheless, we can still cleave to the idea that there is a class of information that, in normal circumstances, is disclosable only with the authority of the referent, and that any relevant rights are the referent's to waive.

Hence the standard model of bioethics gives agents "informational privilege". Also covered by this privilege is that, as well as having all-else-being-equal rights over who gets to access information referring to me, I have a right that others cannot restrict to know things about myself, and to share that information as I see fit. This will be important in later chapters. To iterate: informational privilege itself is indicative of an approach to thinking about agents and about morality that informs the way that bioethics in general gets done. This approach is – broadly – liberal, in that it takes individuals as its primary focus of concern; the mechanism of debate is a matter of balancing the competing rights and claims of individuals *qua* individuals.

iii. Confinement, Unconfinement, Privacy, and Publicity

At this point, I want to spend a little time expanding on a distinction towards which I have already nodded: that between *confined* and *unconfined* information. I shall begin by differentiating it from the familiar distinction drawn between *public* and *private* information.

On the familiar account, private information is information that another person would not know without investing positive effort into its discovery, and to declare information private is to assert a right to exclude others from it. (I shall want to refine this model in the next chapter; but it'll do for now.) Things like financial details or most medical information are paradigmatic examples of information that is, and that it is generally held should be, private. By parity of reasoning, public information is information that others can come to know without investing any particular effort into its discovery, and there is a great deal of it. Sometimes, this is because it is impossible to keep it from others. The facts that I am *this* tall cannot be kept private; neither can the fact that I went to the shop at lunchtime, because it refers to my activity in a public place: though I might ask you not to tell anyone that I went to the shop, I cannot stop others that I pass on the street telling their friends that I did so. Even if I am so wary of people knowing things about me that I rarely leave the house, and do so only at times that reduce the chance of meeting someone else to almost zero, I cannot stop people gleaning and sharing the information that I keep myself to myself. One might hide one's public face, but one cannot nearly so easily hide the fact that one is hiding it.

Genetic information is in some senses like private information inasmuch as that it is not immediately accessible, but we can also say that it is *unconfined*. The idea behind the confined/unconfined distinction is that information about a person is *confined* if by its nature it tells us only about that person. If by its nature it tells us about others, it is *unconfined*: unconfined information "spills over" between people. Genetic information is a paradigm example of unconfined information, because the vast majority of a person's genome, a handful of spontaneous mutations aside, is shared with others. As Graeme Laurie articulated matters in 2002: "the discovery of a predisposition to a genetic condition in one individual often reveals potential risks to the blood relatives of that individual. Thus, individual genetic information can unlock many secrets within the wider genetic family".[29] Information about one's blood relatives is not public – it is not readily observable – but neither is it quite true to say that it's private, since one's learning certain facts about oneself will mean that information about them comes along as part of the package. By learning something about Benny's genome, we also learn something about that of his identical twin brother Lenny.

And, of course, this goes further than Benny and Lenny; we will learn about a potentially large number of other people, too. There is a rate of discount that needs to be applied when we're thinking about other people – it is not always certain that Penny, Benny's sister, will have inherited a gene that her brothers carry, for example, and if it is on the Y-chromosome she almost certainly will not[30] – but estimating the *chance* that another family member carries a certain gene if we know about Benny's genome is fairly straightforward, and so the point about unconfinement stands because the chance that they carry it is itself information about them. If Benny has the gene for an autosomal dominant condition, we will be able to say that there is a 50% chance that Penny has it, and that either Kenny or Jenny, their parents, is a carrier. By comparison, if Benny is haemophiliac, we will be able to say that Penny almost certainly isn't, but that she is probably a carrier.[31] Meanwhile, Kenny might be haemophiliac too, though learning about Benny will not tell us that; and if Penny is haemophiliac, we will learn something about both parents, subject to the small possibility of the same mutation arising spontaneously on both of her X chromosomes.

We can potentially perform a similar exercise in respect of real-life situations such as the one considered in the ABC case: information about one of the parties was, allowing for uncertainty about whether XX had passed on the gene, *pro tanto* information about the other. Conversely, had XX not been diagnosed, but ABC had had a genetic test and discovered she had the Huntington's gene, there might have been uncertainty about which of her parents had passed on the gene to her, but information about her would have been, within a range of probabilities, information about at least one of them. (Interestingly, a 2022 paper suggests that it may even be possible to tell from which parent a gene was inherited without a parental genetic test, even when it is not chromosome-linked.[32])

The distinction between confined and unconfined information is important. The familiar conventions of how to deal with private information assume that it is confined; and though the application of those conventions may require some judgement on the part of the person trying to work within them should another person's welfare be affected by the information in question, they are at least pretty straightforward in the sense that the relationship between persons and "their" information is fairly neat. And though confined information is not always private – what I am wearing is public, but it is confined insofar as that it does not tell anyone anything about anyone else – when information is private and confined and the person to whom it refers does not disclose it, the book will remain closed to everyone else. However, and to iterate the point made a moment ago, genetic information can be private but unconfined. It is private in the sense that, under normal circumstances, it is not available to the passer-by, and special effort must be made to discover it. But it is unconfined in the sense that what a person discovers about themselves is automatically going to give them information about at least some identifiable others – information that, in passing, those others might not know.

For this reason, there is a shortcoming to the standard model of bioethics as I characterised it a little while ago. Recall that the idea there was that, by and large, information is disclosable only with the authority of the person to whom it refers. But the hidden premise here is that the information refers to just one person. Yet genetic information could easily refer to several people, with each of them having at least some kind of interest in controlling who gets access to it and under what conditions. Correspondingly, a person may disclose information about himself, and in so doing disclose it about others: the source of the information and its referent may not be the same. Indeed, there may be several referents. This does not happen with most private information.

A possible response to that would be to say that there is a third category between the private and the public – the quasi-private, perhaps – into which genetic information fits. Such a move has the advantage of keeping questions about information aligned on just the one axis; but the point of the distinction that I want to draw between the confined and the unconfined is that it is qualitatively different from the distinction between the public and private: unconfined information is not just "slightly public". Besides, even if we were inclined to classify genetic information as quasi-private, the normative questions about how we should deal with it would not be made any easier. Whichever way we divide things, the difficulty in deciding who has what entitlements to access genetic information and to exclude others from accessing it, and under what circumstances, stands. The problem I want to confront in this book, that the way we think about information generally does not lend itself to clear application in respect of genetics, does not get solved or dissolved by inventing a new category. But it does rest on discounting the distinction that we ought not to discount between the confined and the unconfined.

iv. ABC Revisited

Having distinguished confined from unconfined information, we can have another look at the ABC case.

Questions of how to handle sensitive information were crucial in the case, and one of the arguments put by the Trust in its defence against the claim that it should have disclosed information about XX's diagnosis to ABC at first instance was that

> [d]octors receive a very great deal of confidential information. It would be burdensome to place on them a duty to consider whether any of it needs to be disclosed to third parties. The time and resources committed to this will be a distraction from treating patients.[33]

Whether it would be burdensome to consider whether information should be disclosed to third parties is a thorny question. The word "burdensome" clearly indicates that considering whether to disclose information would not be just another thing on the list of things that healthcare professionals do, and that this extra task could come at the expense of taking proper care of other patients. This is plausible: time that a healthcare professional has to devote to one thing is obviously time that they cannot devote to anything else. And this may give us reason to think that, all things considered, it would be undesirable to ask healthcare professionals to spend time considering whether and in what

circumstances to disclose information. By having a blanket rule against disclosure, maximal resources can be devoted to patient care.

At appeal, Lord Justice Irwin considered this argument at length. He was
prepared to admit that the Trust's argument did point to a significant concern,
which he called the "floodgates" argument. This argument is a relative of the
slippery-slope argument: there may be any number of situations in which Alice
has an interest in being told something that has been learned by the medical
team in the course of treating Bob, and having to assess the risks arising from an
indefinitely long list of scenarios – whether to tell people of their partner's
sexually-transmitted disease, failed vasectomy, or whatever – *would* be highly
burdensome. Still, he said, the situation in ABC was different:

> [T]here is at least one important distinction between the situation of a
> geneticist and all the other examples given. However problematic, and
> whatever the implications for "third parties", the clinician usually only
> has knowledge of medical facts about the existing patient. It is only in
> the field of genetics that the clinician acquires definite, reliable and
> critical medical information about a third party, often meaning that the
> third party should become a patient.[34]

A very important part of this is the point that clinicians dealing with genetic
information acquire "definite, reliable and critical medical information about
a third party". Genetic information is not about just one person at a time in a
way that other information tends to be. This is what unconfinement means
in practice.

On the face of it, unconfinement might seem to make the floodgates
problem worse, since decisions about even sensitive conventional medical
information will only be decisions involving one person at a time. But in the
case of genetics, we know that the information will concern others inasmuch
as that it is (subject to a discount appropriate to the proximity of the blood
relationship) "their" information too. Thus

> the clinical geneticist is in a different position [from other medical
> professionals]. He or she often comes to know of a health problem
> already present, or potentially present, in the third party, and which
> means the third party requires advice and, in conditions other than
> Huntington's Disease, may require treatment, potentially life saving in
> its effect. One example would be diagnosis of a strong genetic disposition
> to breast cancer. In such circumstances the third party is not a patient,
> but should become a patient. Moreover, in many of the other scenarios
> envisaged, the practicalities of addressing the implications preclude
> effective remedy. Some former sexual partners may be known, but they
> do not constitute a closed class of individuals whose risk is defined by the
> genetic link to the patient, and who, for the most part, will be
> contactable.[35]

However, Irwin LJ reasoned, the very fact that genetics is different means that the putative floodgates problem is not really a *problem* after all. It is a feature, not a bug. In making this claim, he noted the point made by the Joint Committee on Medical Genetics that "[t]he traditional medical approach which focuses on the individual patient to the exclusion of others may be difficult to apply to the use of genetic information":

> For example, testing one person can reveal information about the chances of a condition occurring in their close relatives and providing the tested person with a right of veto over such risk information in all situations may be legally and ethically unsound. At the same time, respecting confidential information is an important aspect of clinical practice and is vital in securing public trust and confidence in healthcare.

And he averred that "[i]t seems plain that this duty already lies on clinical geneticists. There is no basis on the material before us for considering that they are, or will be, distracted from treating their patients by this problem".[36]

As such, no floodgates would be opened, because there is none to open. Clinical geneticists know what it is with which they're dealing. What is important for my purposes here is not the discussion of the nature and extent of clinical geneticists' duties to maintain confidentiality or to warn *per se*, so much as the recognition that the information is, inescapably, unconfined, and that there is no way for professional practice to avoid that. Irwin LJ's having noted that the traditional approach of medical decisionmaking, to focus on the individual as per the requirements of the liberal "standard model", may be difficult to apply in respect of genetics is a shrewd observation, and it informs the arguments that I shall present in the rest of this book.

The professional guidance here points in a way to its own limitations. The 2011 edition of the framework from which Irwin LJ quoted makes a number of crucial statements. Noting that "genetic information is relevant to an individual, [but] it may also be relevant to that person's family because much genetic information will be common to both",[37] and that "[t]he tension between confidentiality and disclosure is heightened in clinical genetics because of the shared nature of genetic information",[38] it describes the dilemma that this poses to practitioners who are bound by *prima facie* duties both to maintain confidentiality and to step in to avoid preventable harm to identifiable third parties:

> On the one hand, genetic or genomic information is medical information that should generally be kept confidential. On the other hand, a result in one person may identify others who carry the same genetic trait and would benefit from regular surveillance and/or prophylactic options. If such information is relayed to other family members without appropriate consent, the trust between the patient

and health professional may be undermined. Conversely, if the information is withheld from other family members, their interests may be placed in jeopardy.[39]

But the way it seeks to resolve this dilemma is at least superficially a bit of a fudge: "The assumption that confidentiality is always paramount is as inappropriate as the assumption that disclosure is always permissible, and the decision will need to be tailored to the individual circumstances of the case".[40] The problem is acknowledged, but little is offered beyond acknowledgement. If one thinks that agents have rights, among which is a right to control access to information, the Joint Committee's guidance will look as though it has missed something important.

The 2017 supplement to the guideline document refers users to paragraph 75 of the General Medical Council's 2017 guidance about disclosure, which says that

> [i]f a patient refuses to consent to information being disclosed that would benefit others, disclosure might still be justified in the public interest if failure to disclose the information leaves others at risk of death or serious harm. If a patient refuses consent to disclosure, you will need to balance your duty to make the care of your patient your first concern against your duty to help protect the other person from serious harm.[41]

Beyond this, though, the GMC does not offer much guidance when it comes to deciding what acting in the public interest would require. Indeed, one might think it outright equivocal on the matter, noting as it does that maintaining confidentiality and disclosing might both be in the public interest,[42] and that therefore "[t]he benefits to an individual or to society of the disclosure must outweigh both the patient's and the public interest in keeping the information confidential".[43] This is fine as far as it goes: there is a public interest to be served by maintaining confidentiality, and a competing public interest in – on occasion – breaching it. But instructing people to weigh one thing against another is of limited use if there is no advice offered about how to set up the scales. How would we be able to differentiate between a good and a bad decision? More importantly, it is clear that the standard model holds sway, and that there is no fundamental difference re-cognised between confined and unconfined information, and so none between how they should be handled.

In principle, there could be a rubric showing how to balance competing interests when it comes to genetic information – though given the range of persons and circumstances that it would have to accommodate, it would probably be extraordinarily difficult to compose and to use (a point to which I shall return in the final chapter when I discuss so-called specificationism). But it would leave untouched the contention that the problems we en-counter when dealing with genetic information are fundamentally different from those that we encounter when dealing with other kinds of biomedical information, because the former kind of information is unconfined and the latter isn't. The prevailing regulatory attitude does not reflect this: it works on the principle that in deciding how to handle genetic information, we work out how we would treat any (notionally) private or confidential information, and then apply that model to genetic information, treating it as a subset of information *tout court*. The guiding presumption is that the information in question is the referent's – the question about whether to inform others is no different than it would be if we were talking about a notifiable infection. In fact, it is not really any different from what it would be if we were wondering whether to wrest control of a person's wealth and share it with others for the sake of the public good. At root, the position is that there is some good φ that belongs to an agent and our actions should be constrained by that, although the wider distribution of that φ without the agent's permission may be permissible in certain constrained circumstances. What is not considered is whether the agent has even *prima facie* rights to exclude others to begin with, or whether the information in this case is the sort of thing in relation to which it makes much sense to talk about *ab initio* rights to exclude others.

That is the contention that I want to challenge in this book. I shall claim that there is no *ab initio* right to genetic privacy, and that even if there were in principle such a right, there would often be morally powerful reasons to override it – which means that it is in practice no such thing.

v. Genetic Exceptionalism?

Assuming that there is something to the distinction between confined and unconfined information, is there anything special in this respect about genetic information as opposed to other kinds of information?

Genetic exceptionalism is the doctrine that there is something about genetic information that makes it so different from other kinds of information that it ought to be regarded as belonging to a moral category of its own. Lunshof *et al* capture the essence of the doctrine when they articulate it as "[t]he view that being genetic makes information, traits and properties qualitatively different and deserving of exceptional consideration".[44] This definition has two aspects: the qualitative and the normative. The first does not imply the second: even if genetic information is not like other information, that does not mean that the difference matters morally and that it should be treated significantly differently from other information in practice or in law. (By analogy, economists might think that we should distinguish goods from services; but there's no evaluative or normative claim built into that.) But things cannot go the other way. If the qualitative distinction is abandoned, the normative must be too.

A normative aspect does seem frequently to come alongside the qualitative aspect. For Lunshof *et al*, genetic exceptionalism implies exceptional consideration; this seems to be more than just acknowledging a qualitative difference. For George Annas, genetic information "is more powerfully private than other types of information".[45] Exactly what "more powerfully private" actually means is a little unclear, but the thrust of the claim is not at all obscure, and Annas thinks that there is something both qualitatively and normatively special about genetic information. At the other end of the line, Bryce Goodman is suspicious of the concept of genetic exceptionalism – but, in setting out those suspicions, provides an account of the doctrine according to which it "sees genetic information as intrinsically valuable, that is, something to be protected irrespective of consequences".[46]

Genetic exceptionalism has a few advocates and defenders, with Annas probably the best known. In the mid-1990s, he and colleagues published a proposal for a genetic privacy law, and a small blizzard of papers elaborating on and defending their proposal, the subtext of all of which was that genetic information is significantly morally different from other kinds of information, and requires special treatment lest privacy be breached. Thus, for them,

> [g]enetic information can be considered uniquely private or personal information, for at least three reasons: it can predict an individual's likely medical future for a variety of conditions; it divulges personal information about one's parents, siblings, and children; and it has historically been used to stigmatize and victimize individuals.[47]

Yet the doctrine of genetic exceptionalism is largely not favoured in the academy. Thomas Murray writes about how the term was invented by a Task Force on which he sat that tried to make, and ultimately abandoned, the case for there being sufficient difference between genetic and other kinds of information to warrant the former being treated differently[48]; and he is just one of the many people to have written against the doctrine's intellectual sustainability since.[49] But academic suspicion of the doctrine does not tell is all that much about its influence outside of the academy: Rothstein comments that while "most commentators have cautioned against genetic exceptionalism" this has been "to no avail: legislators seem enamored of genetic-specific laws"[50]; Article 4 of the 2003 International Declaration on Human Genetic Data explicitly says that "Human genetic data have a special status".[51] This may be partially explained by political concerns: if the doctrine has purchase among voters, then it will be unsurprising to find that it is reflected in the pronouncements made by, and policy decisions taken by, the legislators who are answerable to them. Dalpé *et al* note that most of the participants in their study on attitudes to sharing genetic information in the context of insurance "consider genetic information to be different from other health data. [...] Thus, the majority of participants could be expected to support the position of genetic exceptionalism".[52] Assuming that this reflects the prevalence of attitudes across society, and given that legislators will be electorally answerable to that society, legislative adherence to genetic exceptionalism may not be all that surprising.

Several reasons to insist that we should not think that genetic information is special have been produced. For example, in respect of the idea that genetic information is different because genetic information is uniquely identifying, Gostin and Hodge point out that

> an individual's genetic code is only one of several unique features of the physical body. Each person's fingerprint, hand and face geometry, voice spectrograms, and handwriting samples are sufficiently distinctive to accurately identify individuals with the assistance of modern technology and expert methods of analysis.[53]

If this is right, then there is not much that is exceptional about genetic information. A defender of exceptionalism will interject at this point that the analogies are unconvincing. Sure, the argument will go: all kinds of non-genetic information could tell us something about things like ethnicity, sex, some physical characteristics, propensity to certain illnesses, and so on; but while such sources of information can be identifying, genetic information is simply *more so*. Yet this looks like a set of claims about differences of "degree" rather than kind. Non-genetic information may not be able to pinpoint people in precisely the same way as genetic; but this will not indicate a fundamental qualitative difference – and therefore no fundamental normative one either. And – as Manson and O'Neill have demonstrated – much the same exercise can be repeated in respect of any of the supposed other axes of exceptionalism: whatever is supposed to be all that special about genetic information, and therefore whatever is supposed to undergird particular normative differences, turns out not to be unique after all.[54] (Against this, McGuire *et al* admit that though none of the characteristics of genetic information that supposedly make it exceptional – its capacity to identify people, to ground predictions about their health, and so on – is unique to genetics, these characteristics should be considered *en bloc* rather than singly.[55] But this seems to amount to saying that the tools one finds on a Swiss Army knife are qualitatively different from any other collection of similar tools simply by dint of their being bundled together in a particular way, which is surely false.)

Mention of the distinction between confined and unconfined information may seem to lend a certain gravity to genetic exceptionalism. What other information is like that? However, even this turns out not yield exceptionalism, because there is no reason to suppose that genetic information is the only kind of unconfined information.

Admittedly, it is not easy to come up with examples of unconfined medical information that are not genetic. For example, if someone contracts an infectious illness, they must have contracted it from *someone*, and we can often take a reasonable guess at who that someone might be. But this is not really unconfined information, and not really a good analogue for genetic characteristics: it is one thing to say that Alice has contracted an illness from *someone*, but going further than that is very difficult. On the other hand, there may be a sense in which information about something like Foetal Alcohol Syndrome (FAS), which covers a range of disorders that are caused by excessive alcohol intake by a person's mother during pregnancy, could be unconfined. Suppose we know that Bob has an FAS diagnosis; in that sense, we do know something about his mother, Carol. Similarly, someone who knows that Carol drank while pregnant may be able to make probabilistic predictions about Bob's displaying at least some signs of FAS. This looks to be analogous to genetic information. Still, there are differences: Bob's FAS will not tell us anything about the likelihood of any of his siblings displaying it. Neither will we learn anything about the likelihood of a child with FAS growing up to have their own child with FAS, because it is plainly not transmissible.

Suppose, then, that there is *as a matter of fact* no other kind of information that is unconfined in quite the same way that genetic information is. This will not tell us that there *could* be no non-genetic but unconfined information. That is what matters. Perhaps more importantly for my purposes in this book, there is not a huge need to worry about genetic exceptionalism. My concern is with genetic information; whether what I say translates easily to other contexts is a further question, and I can stand by the claim that what makes genetic information interesting from the perspective of questions about access to and control over it is not that it is genetic, but that it is unconfined. (If I have generated an argument for exceptionalism, so be it; but my position is not motivated by exceptionalist claims.) And what I want to argue over the coming chapters – chapters 3 and 6 especially – is that bringing the conventions of confined, *ergo* non-genetic, information to bear on genetic information will get us tied up in knots. The solution to this is to rethink how we treat unconfined (genetic) information, and then to wonder whether we might be prepared to treat other kinds of information according to *that* rubric.

But before getting that far, it's necessary to do a little terminological sifting, so that we can be as clear as possible about the terms on which any discussion of privacy will take place. In the course of that sifting, we will also spend time looking at some related terms that will turn out to be important in subsequent chapters.

Notes

1 cf Allen, A, "Privacy, Health, and Race Equity in the Digital Age", *American Journal of Bioethics* 22[7] (2022), p 60; cf Allen, A, *Unpopular Privacy: What Must We Hide?* (Oxford: Oxford UP, 2011), *passim*.

2 *Tarasoff v the Regents of the University of California*, 17 Cal.3d 425 (1976).

3 The plaintiffs in the case are identified in the judgment as Ms Tarasoff's parents, which is unsurprising; what is a little less intuitive is that the case revolves around

the defendants' duty to warn *them*, not her (see *Tarasoff v the Regents of the University of California*, at 430–431)

4 *ibid* at 439
5 *ibid* at 440
6 *ibid* at 463
7 *ibid* at 460–461
8 *ibid* at 431
9 *ibid* at 440–442
10 *ibid* at 442
11 Cicero Pro Caelio. De Provinciis Consularibus. Pro Balbo (Loeb Classical Library 447) (Cambridge, MA: Harvard UP, 1958), § XIV. Cicero's claim is that *quod si exceptio facit ne liceat, ubi non sit exceptum, ibi necesse est licere*, by which he means that if it is a special provision that makes something unlawful, it must be lawful when no such provision is made. This is the origin of the principle that *exceptio probat regulam in casibus non exceptis*: the exception proves the (existence and validity of the) rule.
12 ABC v St George's Healthcare NHS Trust *et al* [2015] EWHC 1394 (QB), at 1–2.
13 *ibid* at 37
14 ABC v St George's Healthcare NHS Trust *et al* [2020] EWHC 455 (QB), at 37
15 *ibid*, at 187
16 *ibid*, at 259ff
17 Joint Committee on Medical Genetics, *Consent and Confidentiality in Genetic Practice* (London: Royal College of Physicians, 2006).
18 *ibid*, p 14.
19 Joint Commission on Medical Genetics, *Consent and Confidentiality in Clinical Genetic Practice* (London: Royal College of Physicians and Royal College of Pathologists, 2011), p 22.
20 Joint Commission on Medical Genetics, *Consent and Confidentiality in Genomic Medicine* (London: Royal College of Physicians, Royal College of Pathologists, and British Society for Genetic Medicine, 2019), p 29.
21 General Medical Council, *Confidentiality* (London: General Medical Council, 2009), p 16.
22 General Medical Council, *Confidentiality: Good Practice in Handling Patient Information* (London: General Medical Council, 2017), pp 45–46.
23 Kant, I, *Grounding for the Metaphysics of Morals* (Indianapolis: Hackett, 1993); Kant, I, *The Metaphysics of Morals* (Cambridge: Cambridge UP, 1998); Kant, I, *Critique of Practical Reason* (Cambridge: Cambridge UP, 1997).
24 Mill, JS, *On Liberty and Other Essays* (Oxford: Oxford UP, 1998), p 14.
25 Beauchamp, T, & Childress, J, *Principles of Biomedical Ethics, 7th Edition* (New York: Oxford UP, 2013), p 13.
26 Beauchamp, T, & Childress, J, *Principles of Biomedical Ethics, 6th Edition* (New York: Oxford UP, 2009), pp 45–46.
27 Beauchamp & Childress, *op cit* (2013), p 47.
28 Gillon, R, "Ethics Needs Principles – Four Can Encompass the Rest – and Respect for Autonomy Should Be 'First among Equals'", *Journal of Medical Ethics* 28[5] (2003), *passim*.
29 Laurie, G, *Genetic Privacy: A Challenge to Medico-Legal Norms* (Cambridge: Cambridge UP, 2002), p 3.
30 She might have a chromosomal abnormality, or be an XY male with androgen insensitivity such that everyone *thinks* she is female, or something like that, so the chance is not zero; but it is tiny.
31 Again, there is a small chance that things are a little more complicated: it is possible that the condition arose in Benny as a result of a spontaneous mutation,

and so we cannot speak with certainty about other members of the family; but we can still talk meaningfully about probabilities. This kind of uncertainty will prove to be important at certain stages later in the book.

32 Akbari, V et al, "Parent-of-Origin Detection and Chromosome-Scale Haplotyping Using Long-Read DNA Methylation Sequencing and Strand-Seq", *BioRxiv* (2022), doi: 10.1101/2022.05.24.493320.

33 ABC v St George's [2015], at 13

34 ABC v St George's Healthcare NHS Trust *et al* [2017] EWCA Civ 336, at 43

35 *ibid* at 44

36 *ibid* at 40–41

37 Joint Commission on Medical Genetics, *op cit* (2011), p 1.

38 *ibid*, p 4.

39 *ibid*, p 4.

40 *ibid*, p 4.

41 General Medical Council, *op cit* (2017), p 37.

42 *ibid*, p 33.

43 ibid.

44 Lunshof, J et al, "From Genetic Privacy to Open Consent", *Nature Reviews Genetics* 9 (2008), p 409.

45 Annas, G, "Genetic Privacy: There Ought to Be a Law", *Texas Review of Law and Politics* 4[1] (1999), p 10.

46 Goodman, B, "What's Wrong with the Right to Genetic Privacy: Beyond Exceptionalism, Parochialism and Adventitious Ethics", in Mittelstadt, B, & Floridi, L (eds), *The Ethics of Biomedical Big Data* (Dordrecht: Springer, 2016), p 142.

47 Annas, G et al, "Drafting the Genetic Privacy Act: Science, Policy, and Practical Considerations", *Journal of Law, Medicine & Ethics* 23[4] (1995), p 360; cf Annas, G et al, "The Genetic Privacy Act and Commentary" (1996), doi:10.2172/395 609, *passim*; Roache, P et al, "The Genetic Privacy Act: A Proposal for National Legislation", *Jurimetrics* 31[1] (1996), *passim*.

48 Murray, T, "Genetic Exceptionalism and 'Future Diaries'", in Rothstein, M (ed), *Genetic Secrets* (New Haven: Yale UP, 1997), p 61.

49 Murray, T, "Is Genetic Exceptionalism Past Its Sell-By Date? On Genomic Diaries, Context, and Content", *The American Journal of Bioethics* 19[2] (2019), p 14; cf Manson, N, & Oneill, O, *Rethinking Informed Consent in Bioethics* (Cambridge: Cambridge UP, 2007), *passim*.

50 Rothstein, M, "Genetic Exceptionalism and Legislative Pragmatism", *Hastings Center Report* 35[4] (2005), p 27 (slightly modified).

51 UNESCO *International Declaration on Human Genetic Data* (2003), via http://portal.unesco.org/en/ev.php-URL_ID=17720&URL_DO=DO_TOPIC& URL_SECTION=201.html

52 Dalpé, G et al, "Breast Cancer Risk Estimation and Personal Insurance: A Qualitative Study Presenting Perspectives from Canadian Patients and Decision Makers", *Frontiers in Genetics* 8 (2017), p 11.

53 Gostin, L, & Hodge, J, "Genetic Privacy and the Law: An End to Genetic Exceptionalism", *Jurimetrics* 40[1] (1999), pp 34–35 (slightly modified).

54 Manson & O'Neill, *op cit*, pp 144–145.

55 McGuire, A et al, "Confidentiality, Privacy, and Security of Genetic and Genomic Test Information in Electronic Health Records: Points to Consider", *Genetics in Medicine* 7[10] (2008), p 496.

2 What Is Privacy?

In the last chapter, I made the claim that there is a "standard model" of bioethics, and that one of the things that characterises this standard model in practice is the ascription of what I called "informational privilege". Informational privilege means that information "belongs to" its primary referent, the person to whom it most proximately refers; information's referent is generally entitled to access it, and generally has the final say over who gets access to that information and under what circumstances. In exceptional cases, where there is a sufficiently significant interest served by allowing another access certain information without the say-so of the referent, there may be permissible departures from the general rule; but even then, it would not be the case that anything goes – there would have to be a balance struck between competing interests. By and large, though, informational privilege would mean that privacy and confidentiality were at least pretty much guaranteed.

Much of the language of privacy and confidentiality presupposes that the information in question is confined; but a small industry exists the function of which is to find ways to preserve intuitions about privacy and confidentiality in respect of unconfined information such as that revealed by genetic science. For example, in their investigation into American legal protections for genetic privacy, Ellen Wright Clayton *et al* note that "public policy often involves balancing the rights of individuals to maintain the privacy of their genetic information with the rights of other individuals and the public to access the information"[1] but conclude that those protections are not as tight as they may seem at first to be. Their suggestion is that "[t]he first step to meaningful protection of genetic privacy may be the societal recognition that health privacy, including genetic privacy, is now largely a mirage".[2] Nevertheless, it is implicit in this assessment that privacy rights are at least notionally the kind of thing that the law *could* protect, and ought to strive to protect, even if in fact it does not, and perhaps could not, do so enormously well. There is something there to protect. (It is hard not to sense something slightly elegiac in the phrase "*now* largely a mirage" – a kind of nostalgia for a time when such privacy was real and reliable.)

DOI: 10.4324/9781003312512-4

But what is the nature of the privacy to which we like to think that we have a right, particularly when it comes to unconfined information? Talking meaningfully about how important something is, and how we should act in respect of something, implies that we are reasonably certain about what it is. My aim in this chapter is to test that certainty. (Some writers have suggested that asking what privacy *is* might be less important than asking what it is *for*[3]; but even that functional question does imply that there is a definitional question to be asked somewhere.) If it turns out that "privacy" means something different from what we expected it to mean, or that its meaning is vague, that will obviously feed into claims about the rights that we ostensibly have in respect of it. If it turns out to be incoherent, this might lead someone to think that the very idea of a right to privacy should be ditched. As it happens, I think that there is a perfectly coherent definition of privacy; and so whether or not there is a right to it is a meaningful question. However, there is room to clarify what is meant by the word, and to distinguish it from related concepts such as confidentiality. My final position will be one of scepticism about *rights* to privacy in respect of genetic information – although even here, my claim is not that the language of privacy ought to be abandoned. Certain concepts may have a role to play even if it is only as a shorthand for lines of thought that are more fully developed elsewhere. For example, if we decide that for reasons *p* and *q*, and taking into account the counter-reason *r*, a person's claim to keep certain information to herself is overwhelming, then we could say that she has a right to privacy in this context: the "right" would stand for that conclusion and all the moral debate that had taken place in reaching it.

But I am getting ahead of myself. What is privacy?

i. Entanglements

Wright Clayton *et al* have noted that "[w]hile privacy and confidentiality are analytically quite distinct, these terms are often used interchangeably in research settings and in casual conversation".[4] This seems to be correct on both fronts: privacy and confidentiality are related but different; and they are frequently conflated by ethicists and by lawyers, with the result being either that things that we might say about one are treated as being *pro tanto* things that we might say about the other, or that things that we say about one are treated as applying to the other in fairly short order. For example, Anita Allen describes the American Genetic Information Non-Discrimination Act (2008) as "limiting the use of confidential genetic data by employers and insurers", but categorises it as a Federal *privacy* statute[5]; elsewhere, she notes that that law "aims more to prevent discriminatory uses of confidential genetic data by insurers and employers than to protect confidentiality itself", adding as an illustration that "[s]everal years before the law's passage, a company seeking to lower costs through strategic hiring and retention secretly performed genetic tests on workers to determine their susceptibility to develop repetitive stress injuries".[6]

For reasons on which I shall elaborate soon, this does not look like a breach of confidentiality so much as like a breach of privacy. This is not the first instance in which Allen had run together privacy and confidentiality, having stated in 1997 that "[t]he confidentiality, secrecy, and anonymity of genetic information are major privacy concerns",[7] and in 1999 that "informational privacy [means] confidentiality, secrecy, data protection, and control over personal information",[8] which suggests that the confidential and the secret are kinds of privacy. And, of course, she is by no means the only person to conflate privacy and confidentiality.

For example, in a 1995 paper that is ostensibly on health information *privacy*, Gostin appears to spend a fair amount of his time talking about *confidentiality* assurances and regulations. Indeed, he states at one point that "[t]he breach of confidentiality tort usually requires a special kind of relationship, one in which the patient is able to demonstrate a clear expectation of privacy",[9] which suggests that confidentiality is either the same as privacy, or parasitic on it. In a similar vein, Wright Clayton *et al* claim that "confidentiality, security, and anonymity" fall within the realm of privacy.[10] And the conflation is seen in courtrooms, too. For example, in handing down her opinion in *ABC*, Mrs Justice Yip stated that "[t]here is a strong public interest in respecting medical confidentiality which extends beyond the privacy of the individual patient".[11] Again, this seems to indicate that the conceptual relationship between privacy and confidentiality is, at its most distant, still very close.

From the world of professional regulation, the latest versions of the GMC's guidance to doctors about handling information concentrate on disclosure; but while both privacy and confidentiality are mentioned, neither concept is defined or clearly differentiated from the other. Indeed, privacy is treated as being a part of confidentiality: the GMC's main body of guidance, *Confidentiality: Good Practice in Handling Patient Information*, states at paragraph 68 that,

> [w]hen deciding whether the public interest in disclosing information outweighs the patient's and the public interest in keeping the information confidential, you must consider [...] whether the harms can be avoided or benefits gained without breaching the patient's privacy or, if not, what is the minimum intrusion.[12]

This makes sense only if privacy and confidentiality are the same thing, or as close to the same thing as to make little difference.

I am not the first to note a conflation of what I hope to show in a moment are two very different things. Analysing the development of the law on privacy in England in the immediate wake of the introduction of the Human Rights Act, Gavin Phillipson raised a concern that the opinions handed down from the Bench showed "a marked degree of equivocation between the values of privacy and confidentiality".[13] In this light, consider again Yip J's comment about the public interest in confidentiality extending beyond the privacy of the patient. This claim suggests that confidentiality encompasses, without necessarily being reducible to, privacy. However, she also stated that "[t]he right to respect for private life under Article 8 covers both the right to medical confidentiality and the right to have information about one's own health, including information relevant to reproductive autonomy"[14] – which suggests that privacy (at least in law) encompasses, without necessarily being reducible to, confidentiality.[15] It is possible to reconcile these two claims only if the words "privacy" and "confidentiality" are assumed to be mutually substitutable; if they are not, there seems to be some conceptual confusion. There are doubtless many more examples that could be produced of the boundaries being blurred between privacy and confidentiality. This small sample is sufficient to show that the boundary *is* sometimes blurred, though, and that is all that really matters for my purposes.

Naturally, there are important similarities between confidentiality and privacy, and the most obvious similarity lies in the bare fact that maintaining either will mean that certain people do not have access to certain information. And yet they are not the same: as Laurie points out,

> [w]hile the two overlap in many ways, they are by no means identical. Confidentiality is concerned as much with the protection of a relationship as with personal information, while the invocation of privacy requires no relationship and is concerned with interests that encompass, but also extend beyond security of personal information.[16]

The place of interpersonal relationships in understanding what is going on with privacy and confidentiality is important, especially in relation to unconfined information. This is because information that refers ostensibly to one person may be available to another, without those two agents interacting. The line from Gostin that I quoted a moment ago is compatible with this Laurevian point. Still, there is more to be said. And it is in this light that I shall take a little time to try to define my terms, and gloss those definitions, as clearly as possible. And I think that the easiest way to set out what I mean is to begin by setting out what privacy is not: confidentiality.

ii. Privacy versus Confidentiality

When considering information-sharing, there are normally three "characters": the discloser, who shares the information; the recipient, with whom it is shared; and the referent, to whom it refers. Often the discloser and the referent of the information will be the same person: the patient who tells his doctor about his own symptoms is the discloser and the referent, and the doctor is the recipient. Given this model, getting hold of the meaning of "confidentiality" is actually pretty straightforward. In the simplest terms, for the recipient of information to maintain confidentiality is to keep to himself information that was willingly shared by the discloser. In effect, and in keeping with the etymology of the word, maintaining confidentiality is a matter of the recipient keeping faith. Where confidential information is shared, it is so only according to terms understood and accepted by both parties. These terms may be explicit, but they will often be implicit. For example, a patient and a doctor rarely have to verbalise an agreement to maintain confidentiality; and even when a medical professional lets a patient know that information may be shared with other members of a treatment team, the details can be fairly broad.

Note that confidentiality is possible only when there is a recipient of information: if I keep some fact about myself to myself, then there is no confidentiality to maintain. Correspondingly, there can be no obligation to maintain confidentiality about oneself. In this sense, as Laurie notes, confidentiality is a property of relationships at least as much as it is a property of information. This means that that someone would be at liberty to post ostensibly personal information about themselves online, or on the side of a bus (at least provided that that personal information referred only to themselves). This is consonant with the idea of informational privilege, which implies that information "belongs" to the person to whom it most proximately refers.

Equally, disclosure must be witting for information to be subject to confidentiality. If I let something slip to you, then I have not taken you into my confidence in any meaningful sense; you may have obligations in this sort of case, and I'll say more about them in a couple of pages' time, but they would not have anything to do with confidentiality. Further, the discloser generally has the more powerful position in making this tacit agreement, since she will be able not to disclose at all if the terms on which disclosure is made are not to her liking – although, of course, the power dynamic may change radically once the information is shared: for example, though it is up to me to decide whether or not to tell you something about myself, you might then choose to blackmail me with it. Finally, since it is up to the recipient to keep faith with the discloser, the discloser has the moral high ground.

This general and simple picture can admit of a few complications. In the normal run of affairs, the referent will have the decisive say in who gets access to confidential information and under what circumstances. But though the discloser and the referent will often be the same person, it is important to note that they may not be; and this might matter – there might be circumstances in which the discloser is not the referent and in which disclosure is permissible notwithstanding a background acceptance of the idea that the referent has informational privilege. (The bare fact that a person may disclose information in some circumstances does not mean that they have informational privilege.) For example, someone seeking a divorce will often have reason to share information about their spouse with their lawyer: this would be confidential despite the referent not being the discloser. Naturally, in this sort of case, the spouse would likely know that some information would be shared with the lawyer; but sometimes the referent will not have any idea about information-sharing. Imagine that a schoolteacher suspects that one of her pupils is being prostituted by her father. In this sort of case, the teacher would have a good reason to discuss the situation with a social worker or police officer. Sharing information in cases like this would clearly be governed by norms of confidentiality, even though neither party in this discussion is the referent and the referent may not know about the discussion, and there would be certain implicit restrictions on what the social worker could do with the information. At the same time, the teacher would have an obligation to keep faith with the child insofar as that this is part of the teacher-pupil dynamic; but keeping faith might in cases like this mandate limited disclosure. Confidentiality is keeping faith; keeping faith is usually – but only usually – keeping quiet.

The important thing about confidentiality is that it makes most sense in situations in which there is information that the discloser must have decided to disclose. As mentioned a moment ago, an agent keeping things to herself cannot be described as maintaining confidentiality. In such circumstances, we are much more likely to be talking about privacy (though we may be talking about secrecy – on which, more later). There is a substantial literature on the precise meaning of "privacy",[17] but I shall try to keep things as straightforward as possible: the private I consider to be a matter of privation: of information not being immediately accessible in the interpersonal domain; and to violate privacy is to bring something into the interpersonal, domain – "into the light". (Pyrrho *et al*'s claim that privacy delimits "a frontier between the individual and the collective sphere" appears to be saying roughly the same thing.[18])

This is why I cannot easily insist that information about things I do in public – going to the shop, say – is private. It is tempting to say that the distinction between the private and the confidential is that private information is not shared, whereas confidential information is not *to be* shared – though as we shall see when we consider the secret, this is not quite a perfect formulation. A slightly better formulation is that confidentiality relates to the things that we may do with information once we have it; privacy has to do with how it is that we come by that information in the first place. In this sense, privacy is "prior" to confidentiality, and it is often the default state for information. By this, I mean that most information does not introduce itself into the interpersonal domain: something like my bank balance may become visible to you if you go looking for it, but if you do not, the state of privation will persist. If Alice is prepared to tell Bob something about herself that Bob could not have discerned simply by looking at her, and on the condition that he keep it to himself, and if he accepts that condition, the information would be shared in confidence. If he says that he cannot make that undertaking, and Alice decides not to tell him after all, it will likely remain private.

Correspondingly, if there are rights to privacy, they will be rights to prevent other parties from learning that information by prising what would by default be unseen into the open. A violation of privacy forces something that would have remained hidden into view; in a sense, there is a kind of violence to it. Any duties that correspond to privacy claims are duties to maintain a state of informational privation; but even when we would not want to make an appeal to duties, we could still say that a principle of humility would militate against ferreting out information without good reason. I'll talk more about the principle of humility in respect of genetic information in chapter 7, and it will also inform some of the points I shall advance in chapter 8.

This distinction between confidentiality and privacy sheds light on the appeal to the relationship between agents that is touched on by both Laurie and Gostin, and in respect of which Laurie is entirely correct. One needs to have established the right kind of relationship with others, in which the right kind of "informational transactions" have taken place, to have duties of confidentiality in respect of them: one must have been taken into their confidence. By contrast, privacy may require that we not enter into any meaningful relationship with a person at all. It follows from this that one may have duties to maintain the privacy of persons wholly unknown, and about whom one knows nothing: *coming to possess* information might suffice to demonstrate that a person's privacy has been violated. It is on this basis that we can say that the paparazzo violates the privacy of the starlet on whose window his camera is trained, and (*pace* Gostin) the onus is not on her to demonstrate that there is a relationship characterised by any expectation, reasonable or otherwise, of privacy. There is no relationship to begin with, and merely looking through her window to see if there is anything to see is sufficient to show that her privacy has been violated. (In passing, this allows us to conclude that Parent's account of privacy[19] as "the condition of not having undocumented personal knowledge about one possessed by others", when that personal knowledge consists of facts about a person, must need refining, because though "The starlet wore φ and did ψ" expresses facts, these facts are not constitutive of the violation of privacy: they are only possible *because* of it. She would have had her privacy violated even if the violator had learned nothing about her.)

As I suggested a moment ago, while duties to keep to ourselves information disclosed to us wittingly should be thought of as relating to confidentiality, whatever duties we have to keep to ourselves information that we have obtained inadvertently are *not* duties of confidentiality – and, again, they cannot be, because we have not been taken into anyone's confidence. However, if we do have duties in cases like this, they could derive from claims about privacy. For example, we might imagine a scenario in which the postman misdelivers a letter, and in which I open it before I notice that it is not intended for me. It's a bank statement, and when I look at the balance, it doesn't look quite right; and it's only now that I look at the statement a bit more closely that I realise that a mistake has been made. I have come to possess private information about my neighbour; and though we might insist that I erred from duty by not checking more carefully before I opened the envelope, I would not want to push that line too hard: I do not think that I have committed a wrong by assuming that letters on my doormat are meant for me. Yet we could plausibly think that I have duties from this point on. One of these would be a duty to try to erase what I have seen from my consciousness; and though we cannot be obliged to forget things, it does make sense to think that we ought to let go of certain information to the degree that this is possible. This requirement arises partly out of a respect for the presumed wishes of the person whose bank statement it really was; but we could also explain it in terms of a sense of propriety – of the virtue of not inviting oneself into someone else's "space", and not presuming to erode their informational privilege without good reason. (When Anne Elliot is shown a letter from William Elliot to Charles Smith in *Persuasion*, she is "obliged to recollect that her seeing the letter [is] a violation of the laws of honour", even though the letter is a decade old and – in a roundabout way – does concern her.[20] The fact that the letter is relevant to her means that the restrictions she holds to bind her are much more stringent than any I would suggest; but they are clearly related.)

Granted the impossibility of erasing what we have seen from our minds, I would have a secondary duty to keep what I have seen to myself. Neither of these is a duty of confidentiality, though the latter is superficially similar to duties that I would have had had, say, that neighbour told me about her financial affairs. They are duties of ensuring that, as far as is still possible, the wider world continues to be deprived of the information of which it would have been deprived had the mistake not been made. They are aspects, or sequelae, of privacy. (Should I gossip about the statement, then my neighbour might well lose confidence in me; but, to echo the point made above, the fact that breaches of confidentiality cause damage to the confidence that we may have in each other does not mean that everything that damages the confidence that we may have in each other is a breach of confidentiality.) To this extent, Gostin's suggestion that a duty of confidence may not exist when information is disclosed outside of the "special kind of relationship" in which obligations of confidentiality arise[21] is partially correct – but it does not follow that there are no information-related duties. There could still easily be duties of privacy.

(I have already noted that the private and the confidential is to some extent blurred in English law; and the idea I am pushing here that confidentiality presupposes a relationship between the parties whereas privacy does not is one that is not entirely reflected in law. For example, in *AG v Guardian Newspapers*, Mr Justice Scott had stated that "a third party who comes into possession of confidential information may come under a duty to respect the confidence".[22] And when the case reached the House of Lords, Lord Goff noted that

> (in the vast majority of cases, in particular those concerned with trade secrets, the duty of confidence will arise from a transaction or

relationship between the parties – often a contract, in which event the duty may arise by reason of either an express or an implied term of that contract. It is in such cases as these that the expressions "confider" and "confidant" are perhaps most aptly employed. But it is well settled that a duty of confidence may arise in equity independently of such cases; and I have expressed the circumstances in which the duty arises in broad terms, not merely to embrace those cases where a third party receives information from a person who is under a duty of confidence in respect of it, knowing that it has been disclosed by that person to him in breach of his duty of confidence, but also to include certain situations, beloved of law teachers – where an obviously confidential document is wafted by an electric fan out of a window into a crowded street, or when an obviously confidential document, such as a private diary, is dropped in a public place, and is then picked up by a passer-by.[23]

(In other words, duties of confidentiality may bind those who were not in any particular relationship with the referent or the discloser, because it is in the nature of the information to be confidential. And if this is right, then the distinction between the private and the confidential that I have suggested may not be tenable.

(However, I would want to insist that any duties we have in respect of information unwittingly disclosed to us are not duties of confidentiality, precisely because we have not had a chance to undertake to keep faith with anyone. They are – as I have indicated – duties to maintain the pretence that what *ought* not to have been in the interpersonal domain in which we operate *was* not; they are consequences of whatever duty of privacy there might be. And though some may argue that this is splitting hairs, when it comes to discerning precisely who has what duties and what entitlements in respect of whom, precision matters. Besides, there is a few rejoinders to the concern about hair-splitting. The first is that law – like many disciplines – sometimes uses words in idiosyncratic ways, so the way that the law uses "confidentiality" does not necessarily tell us much about the moral characters of privacy and confidentiality in everyday use. The second is that if, as a matter of fact, law *does* use "confidentiality" in this or that manner, it does not follow that it is *correct* so to do: judges are not immune to solecism. Third, even if legal language reflects everyday language, it does not follow that that everyday language could not stand a little conceptual clarification every now and again. I believe that the arguments in these pages present a reason to think that such clarifications are useful. And even if the law in the end has no use for a rigid distinction between the private and the confidential, ethicists still might. Finally, it is important to note that in the examples considered by Lord Goff in *AG*, it is explicit that the information is accepted as confidential to begin with. That is to say, there is still room to insist that whatever the nature and extent of the duties of third parties, the information here has already been confided (or is intended to be confided) by one person in another. And this means that there is still room to differentiate between the private and the confidential on the basis that the former relates to information that an agent has not shared and has no intention of sharing.)

Drawing the conceptual distinction between privacy and confidentiality does not imply any normative position. However, if privacy and confidentiality are different things, then any duties that attach to them will be correspondingly different; and if duties of privacy and confidentiality are different, the wrong that their violation implies would be different in character, and possibly in severity. Solove writes that "the harm of a breach of confidentiality is not simply that information has been disclosed, but that the victim has been betrayed".[24] I would frame this betrayal as a wrong rather than a harm, but it is not worth quibbling over that here: the basic idea is correct, and this indicates that to violate confidentiality implies a betrayal that is not necessarily present when privacy is violated. Conversely, if there is a wrong to violations of privacy, it is best explained not in terms of betrayal, but in terms of the wrong we would be inclined to associate with prying. Other accounts of privacy see the harm of a loss of privacy as being bound with having lost control over information, and the wrong as being bound with having such control taken away. Whichever of these accounts we prefer – I shall say more about them in chapter 4 – betrayal does not seem to be a major feature. Of course, one may betray someone by violating their privacy, but the betrayal is not constitutive of the violation. Equally, a loss of control over information might also be a contributing factor to the harm of a breach of confidentiality. All the same, that two things have a harm or a wrong in common does not mean that we cannot meaningfully distinguish them: for example, the harms and wrongs of burglary, pickpocketing, and fraud are common, all having to do with the loss of property; and burglary, pickpocketing, and fraud are clearly related species within a genus – but it does not follow that the three things are the same.

Rules that mandate privacy or confidentiality may have any number of exceptions and permutations of those exceptions. As we saw in the last chapter, a general rule that medical staff keep patient information confidential may not require that members of a treatment team withhold patient information from each other; but I pointed out then that the fact that there are exceptions proves only that there is a rule to which they are exceptions. Hence if I tell Alice something about myself, and she tells Bob, then she will have violated my confidentiality – and in doing so, will have undermined my confidence in her. (On this point, Graeme Laurie's contention that "invasions of privacy occur when disclosures of information are made to unauthorised parties"[25] is not quite right: assuming that the person who discloses the information obtained it legitimately, what he is describing is a breach of confidentiality; if illegitimately, the invasion of privacy occurred before the disclosure, and though the disclosure may compound the wrong, it will not constitute it.) If Bob rifles through my bins to discover the information that I disclosed to Alice (or perhaps he is in a more speculative mood, and is simply looking to see if there is anything interesting to be found), he will have violated my privacy. It is fair to say also that Bob will have violated my privacy if he coerces Alice to reveal information about me that she holds in confidence (since he is engaged in the enterprise of ferreting out information that would not otherwise be apparent); and in such a situation, Alice may have breached confidentiality, albeit probably not in a blameable way.[26] That said, confidentiality rules do probably only apply in respect of information that would otherwise be private: for example, it seems unlikely that Alice telling Bob that she saw me on the bus would be a violation of my privacy or confidentiality, since people on buses are publicly observable, and are not taking anyone into their confidence by choosing not to be invisible. To paraphrase Parent,[27] what is inevitably in the public domain cannot usefully be classified as private material.

For the sake of completeness, it may be worthwhile to draw a distinction between "direct", "indirect", and "restored" privacy. I violate your direct privacy when I look through your window, or search through your bins. But recall the claim I made a moment ago that privacy also seems to require that I at least attempt to forget or to un-see the details of your bank statement – and certainly that I have a duty not to try to remember the details. This appears to be qualitatively different from an obligation not to have looked at it in the first place. I call this "indirect" because it concerns duties of privacy in respect of things that are no longer present at hand. Finally, "restored" privacy captures the idea that privacy may be willingly surrendered, but that a state of privacy may re-establish itself under certain circumstances – and that an agent may properly feel wronged in respect of another person's accessing information even if that information had once been shared voluntarily. For example, we might imagine that Alice and Bob are in a relationship, during the course of which Alice takes a photo of herself naked and gives it to Bob. It is trivially true that there would be no violation of Alice's privacy if Bob looks at this photograph: Alice has put the image into the interpersonal domain, and in doing so presumably intended that he should look at it. If Bob shows Charlie the photo, he will have violated her confidence, and – if he does not look away from what he is shown, Charlie may have violated her privacy in a manner that is at least related to voyeurism, since information that would ordinarily not be available would become available. His not looking away when shown the picture would be an indirect violation of her privacy: he cannot un-see what he has seen. But seeing something is not the same as looking at it, and he can avoid looking – and at least try to put what he has seen to one side. Bob, as it happens, does not show the photo to anyone else; but what happens if the relationship breaks down? In that case, I think that it is fair to say that Bob *would* violate Alice's privacy by looking at the photograph, and that he would quite possibly violate it simply by not depriving himself of it (by destroying it or deleting the file) in good time irrespective of whether or not he looks at it. In this case, Alice has a legitimate expectation of restored privacy: something that was in the interpersonal realm and easily accessible could be expected no longer to be. As with direct and indirect violations of privacy, this is not something Alice would have to assert – the difference is that restored privacy deals with privacy that was once willingly surrendered.

There is perhaps something to be said here about the kinds of thing in respect of which privacy rights may be important enough to assert, or even possible to assert. A naked picture of Alice would be the kind of thing that we would probably want to say was private, because people are not generally seen naked; and allowing oneself to be seen naked at a particular time does not tell us anything about any such allowance later on, which is how privacy might be restorable.[28] By comparison, a photograph taken of Alice and Bob sharing a drink at a birthday party would count as private only insofar as that the party was private; and it is not at all clear that she would have any grounds to ask attendees to destroy their copies of the image if she had left and cut her ties with that social circle. This is because attending parties is qualitatively different from intimate situations.[29] Alice may have reasons to want to control the information that she was at the party; but trying to determine what makes some information particularly worrisome for the referent touches on one of the distinctions between the private or confidential and the secret.

iii. The Secret

Recall that Anita Allen mentioned secrecy as being implied by informational privacy. What are we to make of that? I think that there are threads that can be pulled. Though secrecy has things in common with both privacy and confidentiality, it is not quite the same as either. As we shall see, while there is a superficial simplicity to the concept of the secret, this does hide some complexity beneath the surface.

For something to be secret means that it is deliberately made harder to find, rather than merely being withheld from the interpersonal domain. The idea here is that (at risk of reading too much into homophones) to make something secret is to secrete it somewhere: Sissela Bok suggests that "concealment, or hiding, [is] the defining trait of secrecy".[30] She goes on to note that privacy claims are claims about one's "personal domain", and that while these claims overlap with secrecy claims, they are not the same: "secrecy hides far more than what is private".[31] So although there is a great deal of similarity between the private and the secret, one of the differences between them is that the secret is positively suppressed, whereas the private is simply ordinarily-unavailable. (One may compare this position with Allen's assertion that something's being unknown makes it a kind of secret[32]: on Bok's and my preferred accounts, this is not so.) Put another way, we may assume that things are private unless they're disclosed – that privacy would be the default for personal information – but that they have to be *made* secret somehow. That is why a bank statement that I open accidentally, or that you have left in view the table, imperils your privacy, but does not yet indicate anything secret. For it to be secret would require more. And if that is right, Wright Clayton *et al* seem not to be quite correct when, in the course of considering the relationship between privacy and secrecy, they note a "traditional view of privacy as secrecy".[33] Privacy is not a kind of secrecy. And neither is it quite right to say that the secret is a type of the private, because – to iterate – the private does not really hide anything, but the secret does.

Another difference between the private and the secret has to do with the rate at which each is "diluted". Private information is information that, almost by definition, has not been shared: once shared, is that bit less private. The interpersonal domain into which information has been introduced may or may not be extensive (it may just be you and me, or it may be the whole town) and it may not overlap with other interpersonal domains (there may be one interpersonal domain between you and me, and another between Alice and Bob and me, and so on) and so privacy may not be diluted by much when hitherto-private information is shared. But it will be diluted to some degree. If I tell you something about myself but insist that it is private, my having told you at all gives the lie to this: every share weakens privacy, and its really being and staying private would depend on my having kept my mouth shut. However, secret information dilutes only slowly, if at all: a secret shared with a trusted other is not any less of a secret. Information that the spymaster gives to intelligence officers in the briefing room is just as secret as it always had been.

Why secret in this case, rather than confidential? Confidentiality seems at first to fit the bill: the spymaster telling the officer that a piece of information may go no further is in many ways analogous to the patient telling the doctor the same, and we normally classify the latter as belonging to confidentiality. Equally, we may imagine that you tell me something about your financial affairs, and plead with me to keep the information to myself; you are trusting me to take matters no further, which looks to be close to what is going on fairly straightforwardly when we talk about confidentiality. Other secrets may – like confidences – be shared deliberately; and in many cases they will behave like confidences. In this respect, Bok suggests that "[c]onfidentiality refers to the boundaries surrounding shared secrets and to the process of guarding these boundaries"[34]; and this captures the relationship between the confidential and the secret for a good deal of the time.

On the other hand, though confidentiality is a matter of keeping faith, not all faith-keeping is confidentiality. And if we follow Bok in saying that confidentiality has something to do with the boundaries around secrets, that implies that the two must be different. Working the other way, she seems to be correct to claim that "confidentiality protects much that is not in fact secret",[35] but this claim itself really only makes sense if the secret and the confidential are different, and if "confidentiality" refers to more than the boundaries surrounding shared secrets. And so Bok has given us an intimation that we should not conflate secrecy and confidentiality.

One difference is that the secret is better "camouflaged" than the confidential. Maintaining confidentiality is compatible with others knowing that you know confidential information – even with letting them know that you know it – whereas others are not generally supposed to know that you know something secret. (Jonathan Lewis has suggested this useful formulation: that confidentiality is meant to conceal the *content* of the information, but secrecy is meant to conceal not only the content of the information, but its form too – including the mental states that hold such content themselves.[36]) So, for example, though there is an expectation that a medical doctor not share information about his patients with all and sundry, there is no expectation that he should take special measures to obscure the fact that he has that information to begin with. By contrast, the world of spies is not a confidential world: it is a secret one.[37] George Smiley has an obligation not only not to share what he knows about Operation WITCHCRAFT and about official fears that a mole in the Circus is passing information to the Soviets, but an obligation also not to give any clues that he knows anything at all.[38] Therefore far more people may know that confidential information exists than know its content; in respect of the secret, the two groups are likely to be much closer to congruence, and the fewer people know about the existence of a secret, the better. Even the trainee spy will understand that there are certain things that she cannot yet be told, and that her knowing that such things are there to be told in the first place is a little occult. (Of course, everyone knows in an abstract sort of a way that there are secrets held by the State; but it is very abstract: few people could say much about the nature of the information.)

Bok's suggestion that confidentiality refers to the boundaries surrounding shared secrets generates further quibbles. Not all secrets are shared: a secret has in common with the private that it is something that I may keep to myself. But, again, matters go deeper than the secret being a variety of the private. With the private, we are satisfied that information that is not by its nature public will remain outside of any kind of interpersonal realm unless it is specifically sought out. There may be a wrong in seeking it out, and there may be a harm in having it sought out – but that is generally the whole story. The secret, however, is something that we have taken pains to bury. Mere absence from the interpersonal realm is insufficient for the person who has a secret. Indeed, as examples involving spies show, the very fact that there is information at all is often something that we would want obscured in respect of the secret.

Another way to distinguish the secret from the confidential – and, in passing, from the private – relates to the reasons we have not to tell. Bok suggests that the secret is the domain of "the innermost, the vulnerable, often the shameful"[39]; and so for something to be secret, and to be recognised as secret, is for it to be associated with a special reason not to tell.

This is nicely illustrated by the story of King Midas. Among this unfortunate monarch's travails was that he was given ass's ears by Apollo.[40] This was something he tried to disguise: he took pains to keep his ears from the public view, presumably because of the humiliation. His having ass's ears was more than a private matter: it was a secret, and it is a secret because Midas had a specific and positive reason to do more than keep the facts about his bizarre features undisclosed: he had a reason to take active measures to conceal them. Of course, Midas's attempts to conceal those ears (and his shame) could not last: needing a haircut, he had to accept that the secret about his metamorphosis would be shared with his slave. That slave was, understandably enough, itching to tell what he knew. Ovid does not tell us why the slave did not reveal the secret to his friends: it is possible that he feared what would happen to him if he leaked the news, though I shall take the liberty of assuming that he simply recognised that the information about Midas was potentially highly embarrassing. Whatever the explanation, having been let into the secret, the slave also recognised some specific and positive reason to keep the information concealed. Since the slave feared that he would not be able to keep the truth about Midas to himself, he dug a hole, into which he spoke what he knew; but the rushes that later grow on the spot drew the words through their roots, and whispered on the wind the news that Midas has ass's ears.

Does the slave in this story keep (or at least attempt to keep) Midas's secret? My intuition is that we would want to say that he does; and in a way this intuition draws from the way that the information finally gets out into the world. The thought here is that though we might initially want to say simply that Midas took his slave into his confidence, we would be wrong to leave it at that, because Midas's expectation was presumably not just that the slave would not tell, but that he would give no indication that he had anything *to* tell. Furthermore, the slave knows that he will struggle to keep faith with the king, and so his strategy is, in effect, to make the very earth a party to the secret: as we have seen, a secret does not necessarily become less of a secret for having been shared with someone on whom we can rely to keep it obscure – and surely secreting it into a hole in the ground is reliable when it comes to keeping something hidden. The slave is literally burying bad news. Sure, his attempt to relieve himself of his burden without telling anyone comes to nothing; but this is just a matter of gods having a way to ensure that those whom they want to humiliate do end up humiliated sooner or later. A mere slave can't battle that.

Nevertheless, while we tend to concentrate on the possibility that information is shameful when we think about secrets, not all secrets need concern shameful matters. We might have all kinds of reason other than shame to patrol the borders of access to information, and all kinds of reason to try to bury it. I may keep the fact of my lottery win to myself because I think that in some senses it will make me more vulnerable, say by being more open to unwanted public attention and potentially to theft. There is no shame here. Equally, the secret file in the intelligence agency's archive might easily be kept under wraps for perfectly good reasons about which the relevant government need feel no shame: the success of an operation to bring a terrorist to justice may hinge on the information being kept secret.

And yet none of this looks like it is quite enough to give a watertight account of the secret, because concerns about the innermost, the vulnerability-generating, and the shameful might well apply in respect of medical information; but it does not seem quite right to say that that is always *secret*. I think that it would be correct to say that the secret relates to information that a moral agent does not tell, but only half-right; after all, not telling information about other people is the mark of the confidential, and keeping information about yourself to yourself is the mark of the private. It is sufficient for medical confidentiality that it not be flaunted; secrecy implies that steps are taken beyond this specifically to keep information away from this or that person, or from all people. And this extra move seems to have a social element, inasmuch as that it may be in response to, or in anticipation of, others' interest in accessing the information in question. I shall elaborate on this point in a moment, but I need to take a slight detour first.

A further distinction between the secret and the confidential is that the discloser of confidential information is often the referent, and where the discloser is not the referent, is likely to be speaking on behalf of the referent. In respect of the secret, though, there is no particular reason why the discloser should be the referent: when the spy shares information about the terrorist, he is plainly neither the referent nor speaking on his behalf. In fact, the referent may not even know that secret information about him is being shared, or even that it exists. For this reason, a full understanding of the secret would seem to invite another character: the originator. It is up to the originator of information to decide whether or not it is secret; that having been decided, anyone in on the secret is bound to respect it as such. It was Midas who made the information about his aural anomalies secret rather than merely private or confidential by trying to hide it; it is the spymaster who decides that information about the suspected terrorist ought to be hidden away.[41]

More, secret information is often information that the discloser and the recipient both have reasons *to* share as well as reasons not to. Sometimes, they will even have a reason to share it with the person from whom they are trying to hide it. The recognition of another's interest in the information is a part of this. The example of the intelligence agency illustrates what is going on here. The information in the secret file in the intelligence agency's archive is something that the writer (the originator) has – or at some point had – a reason to share with at least some people, or to make available to some person in the future. If there were no reason to share the information with anyone, the file would never have been created, and if spies within an agency never recognised a reason to tell each other secret information, there would be no agency. Some of the people with whom it would be shared or to whom it is available would probably be unknown to the writer. And the recipients of the information would have analogous reasons to keep the information secret. But at the same time, a spy must surely recognise that while there are good reasons not to share information about the operation to bring the terrorist to justice, that terrorist also has an interest in being told about the surveillance to which he is subject. To recognise an interest is to recognise a reason to share information – even if it is in this instance not a reason that we think should be sufficient to motivate action. And so it is often characteristic of the secret that though there is a reason *not* to tell, there may equally be a reason to do so. This point is particularly pertinent in light of the possibility that the secret in the file regards some shameful action on the part of the State. For example, imagine that a terrorist whom everyone more or less knew was guilty of an atrocity was brought to justice only because the clinching evidence was obtained under torture. Here, too, there is a reason not to tell, since it is good to bring terrorists to justice and not to risk their conviction being overturned – but also a competing reason *to* tell, since we may not want to support a system that generates even the right outcomes by the wrong means. It will be up to the agent to decide which is the more pressing.

More pertinently to the interests of this book, a driver diagnosed with irreversibly deteriorating eyesight might try to make this information secret by forbidding others from informing the authorities who may remove his driving licence; and the optician who made the diagnosis would have a reason to tell – and the driver would presumably have recognised this, or else he would not have made a bid to keep the information hidden: the default, after all, would not be to share. Finally, and still more pertinently to the general interests of this book, if someone learns something about his genome and tells his wife, he might say that he is telling her in confidence. But suppose that he pleads with her not to tell his identical twin brother what he has learned, either to reassure or to warn him: in this case, he is not just the discloser of information, but the originator of a secret. Things are perhaps a little more complicated if he does not mention his brother to his wife, but she decides not to tell him because she has inferred that the information was meant not just to be a confidence, but a secret. Suppose she is mistaken in this – that the husband is not really trying to keep the information secret from his brother, but has simply not got around to contacting him. Can she be the originator of the secret? I would argue not: after all, to decide that something is secret is implicitly to say that unauthorised parties may not have access to it, and at least to try to set the terms of who is authorised, and it would not be up to her to decide what her husband could tell his brother about himself. She would not have grounds to complain if the husband told anyone else at all about his genome.

iv. The Taboo

Confidentiality, privacy, and secrecy all belong in the same family; but there is one more member of the family that merits mention, and that is the taboo.

The taboo is analogous to the private, insofar as that it refers to information that is not publicly accessible; and it is analogous to the secret, insofar as that if we have knowledge of something taboo, we are not supposed to share it with at least most other people. However, whereas sharing secrets is prohibited by a person who knows the secret in question, this need not be the case for the taboo. For example, the members of a community might hold that it is forbidden for anybody to look into the sacred box in the temple, even though nobody has any idea of what it contains (or even whether it contains anything at all). Further, like secrets, taboos may extend to cover their referents. The difference is that even when we want to keep some information from the referent, we would not normally have grounds to complain if the referent of secret information discovered that he is the referent. For example, parents might for whatever reason try to keep information that he was adopted from their son; but if he were to find that out, they would not have grounds to say that he ought not to have. This would stand even if everyone is made more miserable by the information coming to light. Equally, the spy might try to obscure the fact that he is being observed from the suspected terrorist; but if that suspect happens to notice that he is being observed, this is the spy's problem, not the suspect's: whatever else he may or may not have done wrong, finding the camera in his living room is not one of them. When information is confidential, or private, or even secret, the referent violates no rule by exercising or attempting to exercise control over it.

By contrast, when information is taboo, and however it becomes taboo, even its referent does not have rights of control. "The central value of privacy", suggests Hansson, "and the recognition of each individual's claim of a protected private sphere can be thought to be justified by the circumstance that every human being has the right to determine who is allowed to have an insight into personal matters or to have access to information relating to that person as a private individual".[42] When information is taboo, there is no such right; and, as such, the person whom the information concerns does not even have the ability to allow *himself* access to it.

The taboo has not, as far as I can tell, received any serious consideration in the literature about genetic privacy. This is understandable, because the context of debates about privacy and confidentiality is provided by a general presumption of informational privilege, and the doctrine (or dogma) of informational privilege would be antagonistic to the idea of taboo information: we take it as a given that, whatever else may be said, and absent some truly extraordinary circumstances, persons have right to know what information exists about themselves, and to access that information. All this is compatible with claims about privacy. We talk about privacy rights, but we do not talk about taboo rights; this is because we *cannot*. A taboo indicates an absence of rights; and when rights are so firmly bound into the way we think about ethics, it is hardly surprising that we find little on the taboo. However, as we shall see in a little while, there are some permutations of the appeal to informational privacy that seem to lead us towards something more like taboo; and this suggests that appeals to privacy rights may sometimes be self-defeating.

v. Moving On

I began this chapter by noting that there is sometimes a tendency in the bioethical and medico-legal literature to treat "privacy" and "confidentiality" and their cognates as more-or-less mutually substitutable. This is a tendency that we should resist. They are not the same; and exploring their differences has led to the identification of two further categories of information: the secret, which covers information that we take pains to hide from certain people, even if they are its referent, notwithstanding that that referent may have an interest in knowing it; and the taboo, which is by its nature information to which nobody has a right of access.

With these definitions in place, I plan over the coming chapters to show that many of our intuitions about genetic privacy must be regarded as untenable, because they actually commit us to thinking that at least some genetic information is either secret or taboo. Secrecy we might be able to live with, albeit unhappily; but taboo we could not. And even if we shift our perceptions and begin to talk about genetic secrecy rather than genetic privacy, we would still have done away with the idea that there is such a thing as a right to privacy in respect of genetic information.

Notes

1 Wright Clayton, E *et al*, "The Law of Genetic Privacy: Applications, Implications, and Limitations", *Journal of Law and the Biosciences* 6[1] (2019), p 4.
2 *ibid*, p 36.
3 cf Cohen, A, "What Privacy Is For", *Harvard Law Review* 126[7], *passim*; Pyrrho, M *et al*, "Privacy and Health Practices in the Digital Age", *American Journal of Bioethics* 22[7] (2013), *passim*.
4 Wright Clayton, E *et al*, "A Systematic Literature Review of Individuals' Perspectives on Privacy and Genetic Information in the United States", *PLoS One* 13[10] (2018): e0204417, p 2; cf Anderlik, M, & Rothstein, M, "Privacy and Confidentiality of Genetic Information: What Rules for the New Science?" *Annual Review of Genomics and Human Genetics* 2 (2001), p 402 for a similar point.
5 Allen, A, *Unpopular Privacy: What Must We Hide?* (Oxford: Oxford UP, 2011), p 157.
6 *ibid*, p 115.
7 Allen, A, "Genetic Privacy: Emerging Concepts and Values", in Rothstein, M (ed), *Genetic Secrets* (New Haven: Yale UP, 1997), p 51.
8 Allen, A, "Coercing Privacy", *William and Mary Law Review* 40[3] (1999), p 723.
9 Gostin, L, "Health Information Privacy", *Cornell Law Review* 80[3] (1995), p 510.
10 Wright, *op cit* (2019), p 5.
11 ABC v St George's Healthcare NHS Trust *et al* [2020] EWHC 455 (QB), at 37.

12 Guidance available via https://www.gmc-uk.org/ethical-guidance/ethical-guidance-for-doctors/confidentiality; accessed 14.v.20.

13 Phillipson, G, "Transforming Breach of Confidence? Towards a Common Law Right of Privacy under the Human Rights Act", *Modern Law Review* 66[5] (2003), p 728; cf p 731.

14 ABC v St George's Healthcare NHS Trust *et al* [2020], at 187.

15 Note, though, how Yip J claims that a right to privacy covers a right to access information about oneself, and on this she seems correct, for reasons I shall revisit in a little while.

16 Laurie, G, *Genetic Privacy: A Challenge to Medico-Legal Norms* (Cambridge: Cambridge UP, 2002), pp 211–212.

17 See Sax, M, "Privacy from an Ethical Perspective", in van der Sloot, B, & de Groot, A (eds), *The Handbook of Privacy Studies* (Amsterdam: Amsterdam UP, 2018) for a survey.

18 Pyrrho *et al, op cit*, p 52.

19 Parent, W, "Privacy, Morality, and the Law", *Philosophy & Public Affairs* 12[4] (1983), *passim*; "Recent Work on the Concept of Privacy", *American Philosophical Quarterly* 20[4] (2983), *passim*.

20 Austen, J, *Persuasion* (London: Penguin, 1985), p 210.

21 Gostin, *op cit*, p 510.

22 cited in Attorney General v Guardian Newspapers and others (No 2) [1990] 1 A.C. 109 at 154.

23 Attorney General v Guardian Newspapers No 2 [1990] 1 AC 109 at 281.

24 Solove, D, *Understanding Privacy* (Cambridge, Mass: Harvard UP, 2009), p 138.

25 Laurie, *op cit*, p 128 (slightly modified).

26 It is perhaps important to note that, though we tend to assume that a breach of confidentiality or privacy is likely to be blameable, the link between the breach and blameability is contingent. It is possible that we might want to distinguish between *breaches* of confidentiality or privacy, and *violations* of confidentiality or privacy, with culpability being reserved for the latter.

27 Parent, W, "Recent Work on the Concept of Privacy", *American Philosophical Quarterly* 20[4] (1983), p 347.

28 Albeit with exceptions: privacy may not always be restorable. Imagine that Alice had volunteered as an artist's model, and that as a result a nude and identifiable image of her is seen by thousands of people. And now imagine that Alice has a religious conversion, and becomes deeply ashamed of her having appeared in the image. In that sort of case, it is not obvious that privacy could be restored; neither the artist nor the gallerist would have any obligations to hide the picture, and art-lovers would still be permitted to examine it.

29 Or maybe I don't get invited to the right kind of party.

30 Bok, S, *Secrets* (New York: Vintage, 1989), p 10.

31 *ibid*, p 11.

32 Allen, *op cit* (1997), p 43.

33 Wright Clayton *et al, op cit* (2019), p 2.

34 Bok, *op cit*, p 119; see also Bok, S, "The Limits of Confidentiality", *The Hastings Center Report* 13[1] (1983), p 25.

35 *ibid*.

36 Personal communication, July 2021.

37 On which point, see Mr Justice Scott's comment in *Attorney General v Guardian Newspapers and others (No 2)* [1990] 1 A.C. 109 at 144 that an MI5 agent's duty "is more a duty of secrecy than a duty of confidence".

38 Le Carré, J, *Tinker Tailor Soldier Spy* (London: Sceptre, 2009), *passim*.

39 Bok, *op cit* (1989), p 119.

40 Ovid, *Metamorphoses* (London: Penguin, 2004), 11:174–193.
41 An interesting observation about the behaviour of Western intelligence agencies in the run-up to the Russian incursion into Ukraine in February 2022 was that they made a great deal of what they knew about Russian movements – information that in previous years might have been considered top secret – public.
42 Hansson, M, "Striking a Balance Between Personalised Genetics and Privacy Protection from the Perspective of GDPR", in Slokenberger, S *et al* (eds), *GDPR and Biobanking* (Dordrecht: Springer, 2021), p 34.

Part II

A Sceptic's Tour of Genetic Privacy Rights

3   Rights to Know and
      Duties Not To

i. Self and Other

Having clarified some of the basic concepts relating to informational privilege, we are now in a position to play around with them a little to see how straightforwardly they apply to the genetic context. My aim in this chapter is to argue that one can tie oneself in knots if one is not careful – but that the requisite care may militate against some claims to informational privilege.

There are two sides to informational privilege: it entitles us to know about ourselves, and it entitles us to exclude others from information about us where this is possible. This second entitlement shows the link between informational privilege and claims about privacy rights. Importantly, and drawing on the arguments of the last chapter, if there is a right to privacy, it implies a right to know about ourselves; remove that, and we are no longer talking about private information, but about taboos. Informational privilege can easily be reflected in law. For example, in England and Wales, and in Scotland, access to one's own medical records is guaranteed by statute under the *Access to Health Records* Act 1990; this right is bolstered by the provisions of the *Data Protection Act* 2018, which also protects the right to keep personal information from others, and the power of which extends to Northern Ireland. Other jurisdictions have their own, similar, laws; and where they don't, it seems reasonable to insist that they ought to.

Informational privilege may be desirable in its own right, but also on the basis of its desirable consequences for decisions that one might make about oneself: for the sake of autonomy, broadly speaking. Any number of examples can be found to illustrate this point. Having control over potentially sensitive information, so that it will not be disseminated without our assent, will make it more likely that we will seek out diagnosis and treatment for medical conditions, thereby optimising the outcomes for ourselves and for those with whom we come into contact. Being able to access information about oneself will also make a difference to the way we perceive ourselves, and being able to control how it is disseminated will make a difference to how others see us: this may well be important irrespective of any harms or benefits that may accrue. Much the same kind of thing could be said in respect of genetic

DOI: 10.4324/9781003312512-6

information as about medical information: of course, a genetic condition is not passed to others in the same way that one might pass on an infection, but information about genes can make a difference to our decisions, and so might be important for protecting ourselves and protecting others, physically and socially.

The twist to this tale is that, since genetic information is unconfined, there may well be other people directly implicated. Information about whether or not someone is infected with a treatable-but-embarrassing disease is not in itself information about anyone else: information about their genome might well be. As such, there are questions to ask about how informational privilege, and any concomitant rights to privacy, would play out; one potential answer may be that there can be no informational privilege in respect of genetic information, just because any given piece of information has more than one referent. But if there is no informational privilege, rights of privacy and rights of access seem to come under strain, since informational privilege is at their common root. What I shall try to do in the rest of this chapter is to show that common-or-garden intuitions about informational privilege indeed cannot stand the strain put on them by genetic information.

ii. Cora's Right to Know

Those who have read the Gormenghast novels will recall that the idiot twin sisters, Cora and Clarice, are obsessed by (among other things) their beauty.

> Knowing that their features are identical and that they have administered the identical amount of powder and have spent the identical length of time in brushing their hair, they have no doubt at all that in scrutinizing one another they are virtually gazing at themselves.
>
> "Now, Clarice," says Cora at last, "you turn your lovely head to the right, so that I can see what I look like from the *side*."
>
> "Why?" says Clarice. "Why should I?"
>
> "Why shouldn't you? I've got a right to *know*."[1]

Because Cora and Clarice are identical, Cora's learning what Clarice looks like will mean that she also learns what she herself looks like. And who would take issue with the idea that Cora does in fact have a right to know how she looks, even from the angles from which she could not ordinarily see herself? In this light, it is tempting to see Clarice's question as somewhat petulant. Either sister's desire to know what she looks like could be satisfied by looking at the other; and being looked at is not a heavy burden. That said, Clarice would have to do *something* – even if it's as trivial as turning her head to the right; and since Cora could learn about her own looks by means of, say, carefully placed mirrors, Clarice's attitude is not entirely without merit. Cora has a right to know how she looks, we might think, but Clarice has a right not to be indisposed; and when those rights are antagonistic, it is not at all obvious that it would be Cora's that wins out. If knowing about herself is so important to Cora, why should it be others who put in the work to allow it? Hence there is already one response to the rhetorical question about Cora's right to know how she looks: whatever right she has may come up against others' rights. Cora's right may win out in the end, but that's not self-evident.

But there is more that we can take from the story. Imagine that Cora and Clarice have never knowingly set eyes on each other, and each prefers not to be seen by the other (or perhaps by anyone at all). This preference looks like the foundation for a fairly straightforward privacy claim. None of us can stop other people seeing us when we happen to be visible, but we're fully entitled not to make visible what would otherwise not be; we may refuse to disseminate information not already in the interpersonal realm. Nevertheless, Clarice knows that Cora, with the right kind of access to the right kind of mirror, could learn what she herself looks like from all angles, and thereby learn what Clarice looks like as well. Would Clarice have any right based in privacy to forbid the delivery of mirrors to her sister's chambers? Or would Cora's apparent right to know what she looks like overwhelm Clarice's privacy claim? Cora's claim to informational privilege means that she appears to have a *prima facie* right to know about her appearance, insofar as that that is information about herself; but this would mean knowing about Clarice's appearance, and so about Clarice, irrespective of Clarice's preferences – and so Clarice's informational privilege would be imperilled. Contrariwise, Clarice's assertion of her own informational privilege would pose a threat to Cora's. On the face of it, it would appear deeply odd to think that Clarice might be able to veto Cora's learning things about herself just because she would thereby become "visible". But this would suggest that, at least in relation to her sister, Clarice has no right to privacy.

Cora and Clarice's predicament provides an analogue of the kinds of arguments that might arise within families in respect of genetic information. Just as Cora learns about herself by looking at Clarice, and would learn something about Clarice by looking at herself, so the same is true in respect of genes. Anything I learn about my genome will tell me something about my blood relatives, albeit with a discount that depends on the proximity of that relationship. Most obviously, if I have an identical twin, I will learn something about his genome. But since most of our genetic characteristics, the odd spontaneous mutation aside, come directly from our parents, I will also learn something about at least one parent. Depending on the gene in question, it might tell me something about both, and about non-identical siblings as well. Or, to make the point in a slightly different way, learning about my genome is a bit like looking at myself in the mirror and thereby seeing something that tells me about myself; but it is also sometimes like snatching a glimpse of something through a neighbour's window, and seeing something that tells me about him. The clarity of the image may vary according to a number of extraneous factors; but even at its most opaque, I will still be able to make certain claims about the things I see. And in respect of identical twins, the window would be entirely clear.

This is not a purely abstract matter. In the ABC case that I mentioned in chapter 1, the father, XX, had – I shall allow – a plausible *prima facie* claim based in informational privilege that information about himself should be available for him to access, but denied to others. In respect of conventional, confined, medical information, the only question to consider would be one of whether the information concerned something that presented a direct and mitigatable threat to others. This would be not enormously problematic. The problem arises because Huntington's disease is genetic, and genetic information is unconfined. As such, XX making a play of informational privilege would appear to be in competition with ABC's claim, formed from the same clay, that she had a right to know about any genetic timebombs that she might be carrying.

One thing that does seem to be fairly straightforward, though, is that there would be no grounds, legal or moral, for the father preventing his daughter having a genetic test under her own steam should the inclination take her. (She might have noticed a pattern of people becoming ill in a certain way that runs through the family, for example. Or she might just be curious. It doesn't much matter.) This means that his right to privacy is always vulnerable; on the assumption that one cannot prevent another person learning about themselves, then the privacy of at least one parent would almost inevitably be sacrificed on the altar of the daughter's having learned about herself.

Over the next few pages, I want to put some meat on this line of thought, and to show that a right to privacy in respect of genetic information is not something that we can take for granted. I shall be using identical twins as a test case, since that allows the argument to be presented in fairly stark terms; but I shall aim to show towards the end of this chapter and through the course of chapters 4 to 6 that the very idea of a right to genetic privacy is hard to maintain.

iii. Some Implications of Informational Privilege

As noted above, informational privilege implies a right to privacy and a right to know about ourselves. To say that one has a right to φ would normally be taken to indicate that one has a right *not* to φ, otherwise φ would be a duty or requirement. (Of course, duties do encompass rights in a way: one must have a right to do something if one has a duty to do it; but we would not normally think of duties as kinds of right and we would certainly not talk about rights if we meant duties or duties if we meant rights.) For choice theorists, the ability of an agent to relieve others of an obligation that they owe to that agent – in this case, my ability to relieve you of an obligation to keep your nose out – is constitutive of that agent's having a right; but interest theorists will be able to admit that though there is more to a right than waivability,

waivability is still in there somewhere: again, absent that, they would not be talking about rights proper.

Hence implicit in the idea of a right to privacy is a right to share information: if sharing private information were forbidden, ostensible privacy would be more like secrecy, and an obligation rather than a right. Also implicit in the idea of a right to privacy is a right to know information about oneself, since not being permitted to know that information would suggest that it was secret or taboo rather than private. Finally, a right to know information about oneself itself implies a right to remain in ignorance; the reasoning here mirrors that in respect of the right to share information. Denying ignorance as an option would commit us to the idea that knowing is a requirement or a duty rather than a right.

A rather different line of argument is available, though. Writing in 2001, John Harris and Kirsty Keywood suggested that that one *cannot* choose to remain in ignorance as a matter of right, because such a right would be incoherent. If they are correct, then the idea of informational privilege takes a hit.[2] Their argument builds on the observation that respecting persons' control of information about themselves is an important part of respect for them as persons at all, and of respect for their autonomy. We need information in order to be able to make anything like a meaningfully autonomous choice, and so to refuse information that may be pertinent to a decision is to erode our own self-mastery in respect of that decision. In tandem with this, they argue, there are certain decisions that might be purportedly autonomous, but that we cannot support from the grounds of respect for autonomy. Selling oneself into slavery, for example, cannot be defended as an exercise of autonomy because it undermines the very idea of autonomy, and it would be incoherent to enlist autonomy against itself. "[A]lthough the sale may be a contract freely entered into and hence 'autonomous' as a choice," they say,

> it is a choice inconsistent with the idea of autonomy and hence not a choice that is protected by appeals to autonomy as a moral principle. Those who deny others the right to sell themselves into slavery do not therefore violate their autonomy.[3]

This claim echoes Mill's position as set out in Chapter V of *On Liberty*: for Mill, there can be no libertarian complaint against governments intervening to prevent someone selling himself into slavery because such a person is engaged in the process of destroying his own liberty, and there is therefore no liberty to protect by non-intervention.[4] Harris and Keywood's next move is to say that, by parity of reasoning, opting for ignorance cannot be defended as an exercise of autonomy, when knowledge is a criterion of self-determination:

> Ignorance of crucial information is inimical to autonomy in a way that other autonomy-limiting choices are not. For where the individual is

ignorant of information that bears upon rational life choices she is not in a position to be self-governing. [...] Of course it is not necessarily irrational not to want to know one's probable life expectancy and many would be prepared to forego autonomy rather than face the knowledge of a looming premature death. However[,] they cannot defend the wish to remain ignorant of a fact like that in the name of autonomy.[5]

To the extent that self-knowledge is a criterion of autonomy, one cannot appeal to autonomy to make out an argument in defence of remaining in ignorance about oneself. And Harris and Keywood's argument would appear to apply to genetic information quite straightforwardly: we would not be able to claim a right in autonomy or self-determination not to know genetic information about ourselves, because the refusal of such information would diminish our autonomy and scope for self-determination.

If Harris and Keywood are right, informational privilege is threatened on two flanks. On one, claims about having a right to remain in ignorance as a correlate of that privilege would have to be abandoned. We may or may not want to say that there is a *duty* to know information about oneself in certain respects, but we would have to say that such information was a requirement of fully-fledged moral agency. (Whether we think it is a duty will depend on whether we think we have a duty to preserve our agency. Kantians might think that we do; not everyone will agree.) The second attack is a bit more unexpected: if they are right, and because genetic information is unconfined, then my knowing information about myself imperils others' informational privilege, because they will not have foolproof privacy rights any more.

Are they right, though? The word "crucial" is carrying quite a lot of weight in the quotation above, and we may wonder whether it would be possible to draw a clear line between what kind of knowledge is crucial (and the absence of which would therefore undermine self-government) and what is not (and the absence of which would simply mean fewer possible courses of action for a nevertheless self-governing agent). And while it is true that having less information may well make a difference to the decisions that one makes, it is not true that it makes one less capable of making decisions *at all*. Along similar lines, Lisa Bortolotti has argued that while ignorance may affect our ability to make *feasible* plans, it does not obviously undermine our ability to make any plans at all; and even if *some* information is a necessary component of autonomy (as when self-knowledge helps us to understand and resolve the mismatch between our vision of ourselves and the kind of creatures we actually are), it does not follow that all information is like this. Genetic information, she thinks, isn't: its absence may confound our plans, but that does not stop us making them.[6] And, of course, people can, and do, limit their future options all the time; but a decision to forsake information is at least in principle reversible.

There is another way in which Harris and Keywood's argument looks a little strained. They are likely correct to characterise autonomy as something that one exercises, and that requires at least the possibility of insight. All the same, they risk conflating autonomous *agents* with autonomously-made *decisions*, and it is possible for an agent to make a non-autonomous decision autonomously. For example, one may make a positive decision not to look at the relevant facts, and to leave decisions to chance. This may be foolish, but it is within the gift of the autonomous to be foolish. It is also qualitatively different from having information withheld by someone who knows that we would not use it, since in that situation we would not be *able* to use it: the decision would not be ours. And so there need be no erosion of autonomy in trying to control the nature of future decisions or by altering the nature of those decisions by filtering some information out; Grill and Rosen are correct to rehearse a Feinbergian argument that autonomy is better understood as a matter of personal sovereignty, rather than a good of which one can have more or less, and that therefore "there can be a right not to know, or at least people can autonomously choose not to know and that there are then reasons to respect this choice, just like any other choice".[7]

Harris and Keywood's line is also in tension with other intuitions about what autonomy requires and does not require. For example, Tuija Takala has argued that to deny a right to remain in ignorance is paternalistic.[8] If we value self-government, then "correcting" a person's decisions, even if fool-hardy and sometimes even if morally questionable, looks to be something we ought to reject.

But whether or not knowing one's genetic information is a requirement of autonomy (and it is worth stressing that Harris and Keywood do not say that anyone has a right to impose information on a person about themselves[9] – and so to that extent, there may be a right not to be forced into what one must accept rationally), there is any number of *reasons* that one might have to want to know or refuse information about one's genome. Autonomy might be among them, but there might be others. For example, one might be concerned that one's welfare would suffer simply through the discovery that one was at an elevated risk of a given illness; but at the same time, one might think that a right to remain in ignorance must be balanced by moral reasons that amount to duties to know genetic information about ourselves: a paper that Takala co-authored with Heta Gylling suggests that "[i]f we plan to have children, there are cases in which we have a clear moral duty to find out about the genetic disorders that we carry".[10]

The claim here goes rather further than that advanced by Harris and Keywood, because the denial of an autonomy-based right not to know does not imply a positive duty to seek information. Yet Takala and Gylling's idea here does not undermine any major claims about autonomy or liberty – nor, even, Takala's other claims. Just as we might say that I have a moral right based in autonomy to swing my arm that is bounded by the location of your nose, the point here could well be that the interests of others make a difference to my relationship with certain kinds of information, genetic information being a good example of this. I would have a right to remain in ignorance, so long as the exercise of that right does not have an adverse effect on others. And even if we are considering something that could affect others – most obviously, if we are making a decision about reproduction – we could still imagine a person asking a geneticist to perform a broad scan of their genome and to make a correspondingly broad recommendation about whether it's OK to reproduce, but still opting for ignorance about the details: "[e]ven if a duty to agree to be tested – to avoid harm to others – exists", Takala writes, "this does not mean that the tested person should, against her own wishes, come to know the results".[11] An obligation to have some sort of genetic test to guarantee the welfare of a future child is not a curb on autonomy; it simply describes its curve.[12]

What is noteworthy and important for my question about this dispute between Takala and Harris and Keywood – and about other similar contributions to other similar debates (such as in the contribution to the debate by Asscher and Koops[13]) – is that its focus is on autonomy, self-government, or something of the like. Disputants may have different accounts of what autonomy is, of how it is best deployed in argument, and of its limits and shape, but they are essentially singing around the same campfire: all tacitly assume that information about ourselves is there for us if we want it, and maybe also if we don't. All these positions can be understood as drawing in some way from the "standard model" I outlined in chapter 1.

But as I have already mooted, the flip-side of a right to exercise control over information by accessing it is a right to control information by denying others access to it: a right to privacy. How far could we push the idea of a right to privacy? Might it generate duties to remain in ignorance when one person's learning about himself gives him an insight into another's genome? And even if it doesn't, does the standard model of bioethics from which the accounts considered so far draw really have the tools at its disposal to deal effectively with genetic information?

iv. The Gerry and Terry Problem

Consider this scenario: perhaps because of a nagging worry about his health in the light of his family history, or perhaps because he is curious and has a little money to spend on a direct-to-consumer (DtC) kit, Gerry arranges to have his genome sequenced, and books a consultation with Emma, a qualified professional who will be able to guide him through what the data can tell him. In the course of the consultation, Emma notices that he has a marker for a particular gene, g, that is associated with an elevated risk of condition C. C does not tend to become symptomatic until around about retirement age; Gerry is younger than that, and is showing no signs of illness at the moment. However, C can cause serious morbidity, or even early death, if and when it manifests. The good news is that there is a good amount of evidence to suggest that a daily dietary supplement, and sticking to a few easy lifestyle rules, can reduce the severity of C significantly, and might delay its onset.

It happens that Gerry has an identical twin, Terry; Emma knows about Terry. This raises a reasonably workaday set of problems for her: would it be permissible to put pressure on Gerry to warn Terry about *g*? If Gerry refuses to tell Terry, would it be permissible for Emma to pass on the information anyway?

It is reasonable to think that there would normally be a presumption against telling, since that would violate Gerry's confidentiality. That presumption would be rebuttable, depending on (*inter alia*) things like the magnitude of the risk to Terry, the possibility of prophylaxis, and so on. The problem would be one of confidentiality because Gerry would, in essence, have taken Emma into his confidence by presenting her with a printout and asking for advice about what it means. However, we might imagine that Gerry pleads with Emma not to tell Terry. This may be for disreputable reasons, or it may be because Gerry fears that Terry would react badly to the news. This would – *per* the taxonomy I offered in the last chapter – shift the problem from being one of confidentiality towards being one of secrecy. Finally, we might imagine a slightly more convoluted example in which the information about Gerry comes to light in the course of some other unrelated procedure, and that (for some reason) Gerry is perhaps himself not even aware of the test's having been done. Warning Terry would, in this sort of case, violate Gerry's privacy (since he would not have confided anything in anyone). Still: some confidences and some secrets might permissibly be shared, even without permission, as might some private information.

However, the problems about what Emma may do with the information about Gerry are not the only ones that need to be addressed. There is a problem with privacy thrown up by the scenario that has not been noted yet. Because Gerry and Terry share a genome, and because genetic information is unconfined, any test that reveals information about one brother will reveal it about the other. This means that Terry's privacy is forfeit if Gerry has access to information about himself. (Michael Parker raises a similar problem, though he treats as a problem of confidentiality what I think would be better characterised as a problem of privacy.[14]) Looking at the situation from this angle means that we have to decide whether Gerry is entitled to information that also concerns Terry. There is a powerful intuition that he is (and I hope to be able to show that this intuition is probably correct) – but if he *does* have such an entitlement, it seems to chip away either at the coherence of his brother's right to genetic privacy, or at the idea that that right is bankable. Working the other way, maintaining Terry's privacy, understood as an aspect of his informational privilege, may well mean sacrificing Gerry's own informational privilege. The problem is made thornier by the possibility that Terry himself may be unaware of the information, even though it concerns him, and may be unaware of Gerry's having had the test. Making Terry's assent a condition of information being revealed to Gerry may go some way to preserving Terry's privacy; but it does so only at the cost of Gerry's putative rights to know about himself. And if we think that it is part of Emma's job to approach Terry on Gerry's behalf, then that means (as Parker indicates[15]) that Gerry's confidentiality is at risk as well as Terry's right not to have information forced upon him.

A further problem would have to do with whether the choice to waive any rights that either sibling has for the sake of his brother could really be said to be fully autonomous. Might Terry feel bounced into giving permission? Might Gerry feel that he has no choice but to allow the fact about his having had his genome read to be shared with Terry? These questions are, however, a little beyond my current concerns, and so I shall leave them unanswered. The important point is that Gerry's ability to learn about his genome is inseparable from Terry's privacy being diminished – possibly with his knowledge and assent, but perhaps not. The closer we cleave to the idea that Gerry has a right to access information about himself, the further we must cleave from the idea that Terry has a thoroughgoing privacy right over information about *himself*. The correlate is that, the more important we think Terry's privacy, the less room we will have to think that Gerry has and should have the ability to access to information about *his* genome.

Whether we side with Gerry's putative right to know about his own genome, or Terry's putative right to privacy, what is at risk either way is a person's control over the information that pertains to them; in both cases, this means that they stand to have lost control of something in which they have a clear interest. Moreover, the arguments that might be enlisted to explain the importance of being able to know about one's own genetic profile – arguments about self-determination, and control over information that relates to oneself – are pretty much exactly those arguments that would be enlisted to explain the importance of privacy or confidentiality. This indicates that, if we care about one of these things, we have as strong a reason to care about the others as well; if there is a presumption in favour of maintaining informational privilege by preserving the one, there ought to be a similar presumption in favour of maintaining it by preserving the other. But this appears to generate a paradox, because we would appear thereby to be committed to the idea that if privacy is something that we ought not to violate, there would be a competing moral reason for Gerry, or anyone in his position, not to seek the information in the first place. Put simply, informational privilege can belong to Gerry or Terry; it can't belong to both. If Terry has a right to privacy, Gerry may have a duty to remain in ignorance about his genome; but even if he does not have such a duty, Terry may be able to present his brother with a moral reason not to have the test, since to do so would imperil one of *his* putative rights.

The question of rights to genetic privacy is not a new one: Sommerville and English suggested in 1999 that

> we may need to reconsider the scope of such a right, which would allow the withholding of information, which is indirectly about themselves, from people whose lives could be changed by it. Children or siblings may wish to access information about family histories – which arguably are the common heritage of them all – in making their reproductive

decisions. The luxury of informed choice should not be exclusive to the individual in the family who, by luck or judgment, is the best informed about factors affecting all.[16]

While their paper does hint that the kind of "autonomy" picture suggested by the standard model of bioethics may be lacking when it comes to considering genetic information, they clearly still think that the right to know comes out trumps; their line is that individuals may have a duty to relinquish too-easy claims about privacy when it comes to genetics. However, while it may be true that to know is better than not to know, this does not mean that there is a *right* to know. On the supposition that the putative right to privacy and the putative right to information are both derived from a more general claim to informational privilege, the value of which is related to its putting one in control of one's own life to the greatest possible extent, the tension I have just identified remains. Arrange things any way you like, and the situation will still be one in which one person's *prima facie* rights and interests will have to be sacrificed on the altar of the other's. Either the right to know goes, or the right to privacy does.

v. The Arguments against Knowing

At first glance, the difficulty facing anyone trying to adjudicate the Gerry and Terry problem is that claims about the value of knowing and claims about the value of privacy appear to be coeval, manifestations of the same basic idea about informational privilege. Seen this way, it is not obvious how one might go about breaking the deadlock. However, it is important to note here what I claimed in the last chapter about the default state for information – and certainly genetic information – being that it is not available: a violation of privacy consists in bringing information to light that would not otherwise be. An implication of this is that learning something requires a rationale that leaving it alone does not. As such, we could imagine asking Gerry why he wants to know the information about his genome. He would plainly need to be able to say more than "Because then I would know it", since to proffer the outcome of some process is not the same as to justify that process. But if his answer were that it is good to know, then that would still seem to be reflected by Terry's most obvious answer to the question of why he wants to maintain privacy: there is an interest served in not being known that is arguably suf-ficient to generate a right of the kind that would be violated by Gerry's having the test. Importantly, though, things do not work the same way in reverse: because genetic information is not by default readily available, there is no onus on Terry to show why it should be *un*available. Keeping things as they are requires no argument.[17] The burden of argument lies with Gerry in this situation, and if knowing for knowing's sake is all he has to rely on, it looks as though Terry's privacy may be defensible. Gerry may, if his moti-vation is bare curiosity, have something like a duty to remain in ignorance.

Indeed, I shall suggest in chapter 7 that an important component of admirable behaviour is a principle of humility, which may recommend that Gerry avoid taking up too much "moral space" – although, of course, the same principle would also recommend that Terry not be priggish about his privacy.

However, it is also plain that knowing for knowing's sake is unlikely to be the only possible thing that might motivate Gerry. Importantly, genetic information may give Gerry an insight into his own health, or his potential future health, and thereby give him an opportunity to do something to optimise his situation.

Granted, there is a few hurdles that this kind of argument must overcome. Suppose that Gerry is currently showing no signs of any illness; a genetic test in such circumstances may look like a bit of a fishing expedition, the justification of which would only be available *post hoc* – a rationalisation of the test, rather than a reason. If that is the correct imputation, then, again, Terry's right to privacy may possibly win out as the stronger consideration. However, even a fishing expedition would give Gerry the kind of positive reason to find out the information that is lacking from the "bare curiosity" account. "Because then I would know and be in a position to act on what I discovered" is more than "Because I would know".

This is true, Terry could say; but it's not *much* of a reason. A fishing expedition indicates that Gerry has no particular suspicion about his genetic inheritance. Meanwhile, Terry might say, if Gerry *does* have some reason to be concerned about what his genes have lined up for him – maybe there is a family history of C – then it does not follow that the genetic information would be particularly useful, since a diagnosis would likely be possible even without it. (The weakness of this last point should be fairly clear already, but I'll spell out precisely why in a moment.) However, this kind of response actually misses the point. What mattered in the argument against Gerry's "knowledge for knowledge's sake" rationale was that he lacked a reason *beyond* knowing it to get access to the information. But now he does have such a reason. That it may not strike Terry as *much* of a reason is neither here nor there: what matters – and all that matters – is that there is something on the "Gerry gets to know" side of the scale that is not balanced by anything on the "Terry gets to veto knowledge" side.

Let that point pass, and return to the idea that the information is not all that important if diagnosis is possible without it. This is often true: a genetic test may confirm a medic's diagnosis rather than providing it. But this hardly generates a reason to veto the test, because a diagnosis of a genetically-transmitted illness based on its somatic presentation is scarcely less informative about Terry's genome than a genetic test would be. For Terry to stand on his privacy would therefore appear to commit him to saying that Gerry ought not to seek a diagnosis at all, which is clearly indefensible. Admittedly, if Gerry is symptomatic, a genetic test may do nothing more than to confirm a diagnosis. Yet it may do more. Suppose that a characteristic symptom of C is a loss of motor control: since more than one condition may have that effect, such a loss in itself may not give us too many clues about the condition from which Gerry is suffering, and so not too many clues about the best possible treatment. Insight into the aetiology of the condition, though, may open up new treatment options. If we know that g, the gene behind C, is associated with a given protein, and that C is caused by a deficit or surfeit of that protein, then we can potentially do something to correct the problem. There is a clear benefit to be had from accessing the information; the reasons to maintain Terry's privacy get chipped away gradually with every possibility for treatment.

But once this point is conceded, it is straightforward enough to apply it to situations in which Gerry is *not* symptomatic, too, and perhaps even to situations in which there is no treatment. After all, it is reasonable to think that prevention is preferable to treatment or cure, and so there is a plausible reason to want to check one's genetic inheritance before one becomes ill in order to take whatever action is necessary to mitigate at least the worst of what is coming down the tracks. For example, *malignant hyperthermia* is a genetically-transmitted condition that increases the risk of death from certain forms of general anaesthesia. If a relative is affected, then one might have a very good reason to get tested so that anaesthetists can be informed, even though the chance that any given person will ever need a general anaesthetic is fairly small. This point stands even if one has no particular reason to suppose that there is anything to find: there might be something as-yet-unsuspected, perhaps arising from a random mutation. And even if no mitigation is available, the chance to prepare is often desired. Perhaps more importantly, granted that there will be time between g's detection C's manifestation, Gerry would be able to keep a watching brief on his health and any medical developments that may help him. Even if C is currently untreatable, it may not always be.

At this point, the prospects for using claims about a right to privacy to stop Gerry having the test look fairly thin. Gerry can admit that there is often a very good moral reason to maintain genetic privacy that is a consideration in questions about who should have access to what information and on what terms, but still insist that this reason is at least sometimes overwhelmed by other considerations.

One possible move that Terry could make now would be to rely on the argument that, since patients do not need to know about their genetic profiles for treatment to be effective, and since healthcare practitioners do not need to know anything about a patient's family circumstances in order to be able to use information, we ought to treat privacy as so important as to warrant a highly paternalistic system – essentially, one in which medics are given the leeway to make use of unconfined information as they see fit, but without sharing it with the patient. This echoes Takala's suggestion that we may act upon genetic information without the referent knowing it, and anticipates the Access-to-Self account of privacy rights that I shall outline in the next chapter. Yet this is a fairly desperate argumentative move – and at least in this context it is fatal to the cause of maintaining privacy, because the principle would apply to Terry as much as to Gerry: Terry would by parity of reasoning also have no right to know certain things about himself, and so it would mean that he was shifting the debate from being one about privacy to being one about taboo. A supposed right to privacy would have been eclipsed by something very different, with which we do not normally associate rights of any sort.

Note also that the nature of the argument here has shifted significantly. When the argument was about whether Gerry had a reason to access information at all, the consequences of his accessing it did not have to be considered. In questioning whether the reason he has is *good enough*, though, this changes, and not obviously in Terry's favour. If Terry's claim about maintaining privacy is still based on an appeal to principle, rather than based on an appeal to the desirability of that principle's outcomes – if it is, for want of a better word, *deontic* – then he and Gerry will be talking past each other. To bring them back to terms would require either a deontic argument from Gerry – and in providing a coherent reason of any sort to access the information that is not counterbalanced by Terry's privacy claim, he has done what needs to be done there – or else a more consequentialist argument from Terry. But a consequentialist argument from Terry would require showing that the good of privacy is greater than the goods that accrue from knowledge, which is no easy task; and it would mean abandoning the idea of an *ab initio* right to privacy, since the "right" would only ever be a function of what is most desirable all things considered. Either way, Terry's claim that he has a right to privacy looks to be increasingly unsustainable.

The one remaining respect in which Terry might have some slender hope of undermining Gerry's rationale for accessing genetic information, and thereby maintaining the relative normative power of his claimed right to genetic privacy, is based on a dispute about the prognostic power of genetic data should Gerry currently be asymptomatic. Essentially, the argument works – if it works – on two fronts, though both capitalise on the trivial points that prognosis is by definition a matter of predictions about the future, that the future is an uncertain business, and that a test that reveals the presence of a certain gene or marker does not mean that the condition with which it is associated will manifest.

On the first front, this is because becoming ill and potentially dying from an illness to which we are genetically susceptible requires that we do not die of any other thing long before our genes have had a chance to work their dubious magic, and there is always a non-zero chance that we will; the relative importance of revealing information ought to be discounted by these considerations. At the same time, the importance of privacy does not have that kind of discount applied to it: its value applies here and now and indefinitely into the future. On the second, even if we ignore all the other things that might kill us, carrying a gene associated with a given condition does not necessarily provide a reliable guide to the future. Many illnesses are multifactorial, so the presence of a gene may increase the likelihood of that illness manifesting, but it in no way guarantees it. Left here, that point is grist to Gerry's mill: if there is a lifestyle alteration he can make in order to head off whatever is coming down the genetic track towards him, then knowing about his genome would be very useful. However, Terry might continue to point out that his point stands in respect even of conditions that are monofactorial. Strachan and Read write that "[b]y definition, a dominant character[18] is manifested in a heterozygous person, and so should show 100% pentrace". But, they continue,

> [m]any human characters, although generally showing dominant inheritance, occasionally skip a generation. [...] This would be described as a case of non-penetrance.

> There is no mystery about non-penetrance – indeed, 100% penetrance is the more surprising phenomenon. Very often the presence or absence of a character depends, in the main and in normal circumstances, on the genotype at one locus, but an unusual genetic background, a particular lifestyle, or maybe just chance means that the occasional person may fail to manifest the character.[19]

Relatedly, some genes have variable expression: a given gene may announce its presence in a number of ways, or not at all, depending on the other genes that a person carries, or on the environment, or on blind luck.[20] Therefore, we might legitimately expect the strength of a claim about a right to know to be modified by the likelihood of the gene actually doing anything. Once again, privacy is not subject to any such statistical discounting: it doesn't make sense to raise questions about the likelihood of the privilege that a right to privacy reflects doing anything, or when it would do it. Assuming that the naïve accounts of Gerry's right to know and Terry's right to privacy are plausible and each has a roughly equal initial appeal, the fact that Gerry's interest in knowing can be discounted and Terry's cannot seems to count in favour of maintaining Terry's privacy.

But for Terry to argue like this would be pretty last-ditch. Even if genes are only imperfectly predictive, the fact stands that they have predictive power, and that knowing that there is a chance of this or that happening to us within a tolerably definable time-period is plausibly a good in itself, as well as being a prerequisite of realising other goods. If Terry does have a right to privacy, it seems to be a right of only the most formalistic sort; but – if the strategy chosen to resolve the problem is consequentialist – he may not have any such right at all.

A further important point in all this is that even if our normative assessment of Terry's position spins out the other way, and we decide that he does have a bankable right to privacy such that others, including his brother, may not engage in activities the outcome of which would be to reveal information about his genome, *this also puts the idea of genetic privacy at risk* by undermining the idea of informational privilege: an agent no longer has authority over access to "his own" genome. And since the idea of genetic privacy relies on that authority, Terry should perhaps be careful what he wishes for. If the referent of information does not have rights to access to it, that information is not private: it is taboo. Gerry and Terry might be on good terms, and agree that it's a taboo that it would be permissible or even desirable to break; but the point would stand that we would no longer be talking about privacy. And so while the picture I have been painting over the past few pages – one in which Terry probably does not have a right to privacy – is very different from the picture I painted in the 2011 paper that is this chapter's ancestor, in which I suggested that Gerry might have a duty to remain in ignorance,[21] there is a fundamental consonance between them. Shake things up however one will: informational privilege is in trouble.

vi. Who Violates Privacy?

The argument above suggests that even if Terry could mount a claim about genetic privacy that would be sufficient to give Gerry *a reason* not to have the test, it will not suffice to show that it is wrong for him to have it. In effect, claims about rights not withstanding, it would be permissible for him to have violated Terry's privacy. But we could go even further and say that, even though Terry's putative privacy right has been eroded, this is not something we can pin on Gerry in any morally weighty sense. Such a claim is built around a version of the doctrine of double effect (DDE). Most commonly associated with end-of-life questions, the DDE promises to provide a way to think about the administration of certain drugs to minimise distress, even though they may shorten life. The doctrine can be expounded in a few steps:

> When the administration of a standard dose of analgesia by A to a patient B to relieve B's discomfort at the end of life is predicted to accelerate B's death, such administration is not an instance of A killing B, provided that:
>
> 1   the shortening of life is a foreseen but not intended consequence of its administration, and
> 2   the acceleration of death is not the means by which suffering is relieved.

What is central to the doctrine is the idea that A can have acted in such a way as to accelerate the end of B's life without necessarily having killed B; and if B was killed, it was not by A. It is possible to add to that a claim about permissibility, such that actions that may accelerate B's death may be *permissible* provided that those actions are ordinarily permissible: since administering a standard dose of analgesia is obviously permissible, then administering it in these conditions is more likely to be permissible as well. If the action is wrong, it is not wrong just because it is killing.

The DDE can be coopted into the Gerry and Terry problem, in which case it would look something like this:

> When the pursuit of information about his own genome by Gerry is predicted to reveal otherwise private information about Terry, such a pursuit is not an instance of Gerry violating Terry's privacy, provided that:
>
> 1 revealing the information about Terry is a foreseen but not intended consequence Gerry's action, and
> 2 revealing otherwise private information about Terry's is not the means by which Gerry obtains information about his own genome.

Condition (2) probably needs a bit of elaboration: when it comes to it, it means that there is a difference between Gerry's finding out about Terry's genome thanks to a blood test that he himself has taken, and his finding out about Terry's genome by (say) tricking Terry into having a blood test, or by rifling through his medical records. And as with the end-of-life version of the doctrine, we can append a claim about permissibility, along the lines that there would be nothing impermissible about Gerry's taking a test to find out about his own genome, even though Terry's privacy would be forfeit, provided that finding out about one's own genome is ordinarily permissible. But, again, the important point would be that we could admit that Terry's privacy has been violated, without having to admit that its violation is morally attributable to Gerry. And as such, Terry would have no right that is bankable against Gerry.

Clearly, a lot would ride on accepting a version of the DDE, and believing that there can be a foreseen but unintended consequence of an intended act. If one rejects the doctrine, then this defence of Gerry's test will be a nonstarter. Nevertheless, it does capture the intuition that that there is something morally different between Gerry's having taken a blood test, and his having looked at his brother's medical records – and that the latter is potentially more blameable than the former. Yet if it is more blameable, it must be the case that there is a difference between them, since while things might be morally alike and yet different by their nature, it is harder for them to be alike by their nature yet morally different. The doctrine helps clarify what that difference might be.

Once again, we may want to bite the bullet and insist that the intuition is misplaced, and that there really is no difference between taking a test and looking at medical records, since the effective result is the same. This is a perfectly respectable position to adopt – but it does little to preserve the idea of genetic privacy because, once again, it would involve denying informational privilege, the foundation upon which claims about genetic privacy are built.

vii. What Follows?

Maybe we think that Terry does not after all have a right to privacy over his genome. Maybe we think the opposite, and that he *does* have such a right, and that Gerry has a duty to remain in ignorance. A lot of information is available to Gerry without a genetic test, after all.

But this is compatible with thinking that, however we settle it, the scenario outlined in the Gerry and Terry problem is exceptional, because each is one of a pair of monozygotic twins. Whatever solution to the problem we settle on might provide us with nothing particularly generalisable to say about genetic information and rights to control information about one's own genome. Perhaps the Gerry and Terry problem amounts to an amusing little mind game that we might play while thinking about a small number of policies that would apply in the real world, but nothing more.

This is an argumentative strategy that we would do well not to pursue, for at least five reasons. The first, and the most important, is that the Gerry and Terry problem is not actually exceptional. Making our protagonists identical twins puts the problem into bright primary colours, but it is a problem that, in slightly more muted shades, appears for anyone else. Genetic information about one person can tell us about family members other than identical twins. Hence while information about mothers, fathers, and fraternal siblings cannot be inferred directly from a person's genome, implications can still be drawn. As such, the Gerry and Terry problem at least throws into relief a problem that is pervasive.

The second is that, rare as they may be, the real world does contain identical twins; and so to discount scenarios involving them as mere thought experiments is to store up problems when we try to apply our principles to the real world. (At the very least, there would be an unmet need to account for those situations in which we are dealing with identical twins.) The third follows fairly closely from this, and it is that it seems to be pushing the limits of moral luck a bit far to suppose that a person like Gerry or Terry may in *principle* have fewer informational entitlements or less informational privilege – whether that be to access to information or to privacy in respect of that information – than someone like Emma just because of the fact that they have an identical twin and Emma doesn't. The fourth is that, by making an exception of monozygotic twins, we are forced to increase the world's stock of moral rules and the arguments on which they rely *ad hoc*. And the fifth – though, to my mind, the second most important – is that it is bad philosophical practice to shape our principles according to the outcomes that we want to maintain or in order to preserve a set of intuitions about privacy and access to information.

There may be more reasons not to pursue the strategy. Five is plenty for my purposes. That said, it would pay us to retrace our steps for a moment to elucidate the third point.

I take it as an axiom of any plausible system of moral philosophy that, once we recognise that someone is a moral agent, they have the same moral gravity as any other moral agent, irrespective of the contingencies of their life. Gerry and Terry are the moral equals of each other, and of everyone else. But while moral equality requires equality of consideration, it does not require sameness of treatment. Treating people *as equals* is compatible with treating them differently in certain respects and in at least some circumstances; and different treatment may be not only warranted but required on occasion. It is not difficult to establish the truth of this assertion: Dworkin's example of deciding how much of a lifesaving drug to allocate to the ill child and the healthy child suffices.[22] And therefore it is possible that we should treat Gerry (or Terry) differently from how we treat any other person, not because of who he is, but because of relevant facts about his situation.

What would remain to be shown is that his situation really is different in a morally-relevant way. It is not at all clear to me that simply being an identical twin is sufficient to make the kind of moral difference that would mean that some people are allowed to exclude all others from information about their genomes while Terry is not (or, if we think that Terry's right to privacy is the more important, that some people are allowed to know their genetic inheritance while Gerry is not). All else being equal, all of the rationales that we might present for any other person having access to her genetic information, or the right to deny others access, would appear to apply to Gerry and Terry. Furthermore, there would be a problem of policing the boundaries. Imagine for a moment Gerry and Terry have a sister: call her Cherry. Obviously, her genome will differ in some ways from her brothers'. In other ways, it will be very similar – similar enough for her knowledge of her own genome to give her knowledge of her brothers', and *vice versa*. What would that mean for Cherry's informational privilege, though? Given that there will be differences between her genome and her brothers', how should we assess the weight of her claim to know information about herself and to prevent others from knowing it? Perhaps the idea might be that her right to know her information ought to be weighed relative to the amount of her genome that she has in common. I shall arc back to this idea in chapter 6.

A more radical response is to suggest that we should abandon looking for a solution and aim for dissolution instead. The problem itself is unavoidable, the thought might go, because grounding our arguments in appeals to autonomy and the stake that a person has in this or that information being more or less well known is to subscribe to the individualistic picture of moral agency upon which the standard model of bioethics is built but that is unsustainable in respect of genetics, given that genetics is by its nature transpersonal and genetic information is unconfined. If individualistic arguments don't fit the moral reality, it oughtn't to be a surprise that we'll end up tied in knots; therefore we perhaps ought to ditch the arguments. As we shall see later in this book, there is something in this that I think we should take seriously; but taken too broadly, it seems like a counsel of despair – and one that does nothing more than reverse the problem: if neither Gerry nor Terry has any informational privilege, we'd still be no wiser when it comes to knowing what to do when their desires are incompatible.

However, this last suggestion does contain within itself the seeds of the next step in the argument. The assumption that was made throughout the last chapter was that there is – all things being equal – a right to privacy over genetic information. That right may be threatened by particular circumstances, but the problem is one of what to do *given* a right to privacy, and *given* circumstances that nibble away at it. This assumption chimes nicely with what I suspect is a lot of people's intuitions, and it resonates with the professional guidance I considered in chapter 1, the emphasis on which is universally that information should be kept under wraps unless there are very good extenuating reasons.[23] Still, this does leave open the question of whether the very idea of a right to privacy is all that applicable to genetic information after all. In the coming chapters, I shall present my reasons for thinking that it may not be: at least, not straightforwardly.

So as a precursor to decisions about whether and when it is permissible to violate a person's putative privacy rights, it is worth spending some time on a more fundamental question: what is a privacy right, and how would it be applied to genetic information, to begin with? It is to that question that I shall turn my attention in the next chapter.

Notes

1 Peake, M, *Titus Groan*, repr. in *The Gormenghast Trilogy* (London: Vintage, 1999), p 278 (slightly modified).
2 Harris, J, & Keywood, K, "Ignorance, Information and Autonomy", *Theoretical Medicine and Bioethics* 22[5] (2001), pp 415–436.
3 *ibid*, p 420.
4 Mill, JS, *On Liberty and Other Essays* (Oxford: Oxford UP, 1998), p 114.
5 Harris & Keywood, *op cit*, p 421.
6 Bortolotti, L, "The Relative Importance of Undesirable Truths", *Medicine, Health Care, and Philosophy* 16[4] (2013), *passim*.
7 Grill, K, & Rosen, A, "Healthcare Professionals' Responsibility for Informing Relatives at Risk of Hereditary Disease", *Journal of Medical Ethics* 47[12] (2021): e12, p 4.
8 Takala, T, "Genetic Ignorance and Reasonable Paternalism", *Theoretical Medicine and Bioethics* 22[5] (2001), p 490.
9 Harris & Keywood, *op cit*, p 432.
10 Takala, T, & Gylling, H, "Who Should Know about Our Genetic Makeup and Why?" *Journal of Medical Ethics* 26[3] (2000), p 172.
11 Takala, T, *op cit*, p 486.
12 There is, of course, an enormous literature dealing with whether it is possible to harm or benefit merely potential people, which I shall deliberately leave entirely to one side for the sake of this argument.

13 Asscher, E, & Koops, B-J, "The Right Not to Know and Preimplantation Genetic Diagnosis for Huntington's Disease", *Journal of Medical Ethics* 36[1] (2010), pp 30–33.

14 Parker, M, "Genetics and the Interpersonal Elaboration of Ethics", *Theoretical Medicine and Bioethics* 22[5] (2001), p 453 and *passim*.

15 *ibid*, p 452.

16 Sommerville, A, & English, V, "Genetic Privacy: Orthodoxy or Oxymoron?" *Journal of Medical Ethics* 25[2] (1999), pp 144–150, p 150.

17 To deny this is to fall into a version of the trap of what I have elsewhere called *hyperpositivism*: the fallacy of thinking that a (negative) decision not to φ must be characterised a (positive) decision to ψ (see Brassington, 2020, p 10). More broadly, hyperpositivism would be the fallacy of thinking that the absence of some φ (or the absence of a need for some φ) must be characterised as the presence of ψ (or the presence of a need for ψ) – in this case, of thinking that we need a positive reason to leave things be in addition to a negative reason not to interfere.

18 At p 62, the authors clarify that characters are the observable properties of an organism, though observability may only be possible through laboratory analysis. For my purposes, I shall not differentiate between "character" and "characteristic".

19 Strachan, T, & Read, A, *Human Molecular Genetics, 4th Edition* (New York: Garland Science, 2011), p 73.

20 *ibid*, p 74.

21 Brassington, I, "Is There a Duty to Remain in Ignorance?" 32[2] (2011), pp 101–115, *passim*.

22 Dworkin, R, *Taking Rights Seriously* (London: Bloomsbury, 2013); cf Nagel, T, "The Justification of Equality", *Crítica: Revista Hispanoamericana de Filosofía* 10[28] (1978), *passim*.

23 That the guidance often considers matters in terms of confidentiality rather than privacy, or conflates the two, does not matter at this point.

4   What Is a Privacy Right?

i. Privacy and Privacy Rights

The argument of the last chapter depended on taking as a starting point that there is such a thing as informational privilege, manifested as the complementary rights to privacy and to know about oneself. On this model, and all else being equal, the referent of a given piece of information can exclude others from access to it because of his or her privileged status in respect of it. But as we saw, there may be anomalies and paradoxes thrown up by this kind of model. They may be confined to situations such as the Gerry and Terry case, when for some reason all is not equal; but they may also refer to something a bit deeper. After all, it would seem not to be to the credit of our intuitions about informational privilege that they should be confoundable at all.

But, beyond its being an aspect of informational privilege, what is the nature of a putative right to privacy? The "privacy" bit was dealt with in chapter 2, and though Daniel Solove may be correct in his suggestion that seeking a precise definition is a fool's errand – for him, the word "privacy" is possible to understand in a range of ways that resemble each other but that never coalesce into a precise definition[1] – I believe that enough was done there to give us a general grasp on the concept. But it remains to be seen quite what a *right* to privacy is. We tend to assume that there is one, that it is a *datum* of moral debate – that is, it is something that we can bring to the table when we are talking about what agents may or may not do – and that it is important. Admittedly, we could maintain at least most of our attitudes about a putative right to privacy for most of the time without letting the precise nature of the right worry us too much. But this is arguably because rights are not things we need to think about most of the time at all. When a practical problem about access to and control of genetic information arises, though, it seems reasonable to assume that having an account of the nature of the rights that may be in question would be useful. Correspondingly, if it turns out that a "right to genetic privacy" means something different from what we expected it to mean, or that its meaning is vague, then it might be that this would force us to reevaluate certain intuitions about who has or ought to have access to what information, and on what terms. Accordingly, what I intend to do in this chapter is to present a brief survey of

DOI: 10.4324/9781003312512-7

the ways in which a right to privacy tends to be conceptualised, and to consider how well they might apply to genetic information. If none of the conceptualisations applies easily – as I think will turn out to be the case – there will be a number of possible conclusions to draw. We might think that a theory of privacy rights that does not apply to every situation in which we would expect there to be a privacy right is false; it would follow from this that if no theory applies to genetic information, genetic information is a possible confounder to the very idea of privacy rights. We might think, more conservatively, that the non-applicability of the theories to genetic information means simply that there is no such thing as an *ab initio* right to *genetic* privacy, but leave aside other areas. Or we might think that there is such a thing as a right to genetic privacy, and that the failure of extant theories to account for it simply shows that we need a new one. This last option has a whiff of dogmatism about it. The middle option is more attractive, and it is the one I shall orbit in the remainder of this book. But first, I have to explain why.

ii. Kinds of Privacy Right

In his 2002 survey, Solove identifies six potential ways to understand what a privacy right would entail: being let alone; limiting access to the self; secrecy; control over personal information; personhood; and intimacy. The later ways named by Solove strike me as being either derivative or developments of the first, and so it is with a right to privacy as a right to be let alone that I shall begin. However, there is a little more preparatory whittling that we can do. Secrecy is, on the grounds I have articulated in chapter 2, different from privacy, and so excluded as a candidate way to understand privacy and privacy rights; personhood and intimacy are also excluded, on the grounds that while either may generate reasons to respect privacy, neither will explain it as a right; furthermore, we can state from the off that intimacy's relationship with *genetic* privacy is tenuous at best. I do not intend in what follows to go all that deeply into the different ways in which privacy may be understood – rather, my concern is to give a sense of the lie of the land, with the intention of trying to get to grips with what each conceptualisation might mean for genetic information.

(a) Privacy as the Right to Be Let Alone

Solove follows many other authors in tracing the idea of a privacy right as a right to be let alone back to the nineteenth century, and to Warren and Brandeis' attempt to formulate a right to privacy in law. Writing in 1890, their concern was motivated by the perceived threat to privacy presented by the popular press and such technologies as the portable camera:

> Instantaneous photographs and newspaper enterprise have invaded the sacred precincts of private and domestic life; and numerous mechanical

devices threaten to make good the prediction that 'what is whispered in the closet shall be proclaimed from the house-tops.' For years there has been a feeling that the law must afford some remedy for the unauthorized circulation of portraits of private persons; and the evil of the invasion of privacy by the newspapers, long keenly felt, has been but recently discussed by an able writer. [...] To satisfy a prurient taste the details of sexual relations are spread broadcast in the columns of the daily papers. To occupy the indolent, column upon column is filled with idle gossip, which can only be procured by intrusion upon the domestic circle.[2]

That they took as read that there is something for which the law ought to provide remedy serves to indicate their belief in a right to privacy that is not the entire creation of the law. The importance of protecting private individuals from prurient "intrusion upon the domestic circle" was linked to a particular conception of flourishing:

The intensity and complexity of life, attendant upon advancing civilization, have rendered necessary some retreat from the world, and man, under the refining influence of culture, has become more sensitive to publicity, so that solitude and privacy have become more essential to the individual; but modern enterprise and invention have, through invasions upon his privacy, subjected him to mental pain and distress, far greater than could be inflicted by mere bodily injury.[3]

This passage helps make clear that a right to privacy was, under this conception, a right to be let alone. (This doctrine has had a wide influence: for example, it is cited with approval by Justice Stewart in *Roe v Wade*.[4]) For the sake of ease over the coming pages, I shall call this kind of account, in which the right to be let alone is key, the "RLA account".

An interesting detail of the argument that Warren and Brandeis put is that there is a long tradition of thinking that a human divorced from other humans was vulnerable to losing his humanity entirely. Aristotle had thought that humans were social by nature, that the formation of the state reflects this, and that someone stateless by nature must be either a beast or a god[5]; Bradley had echoed this in 1876 when he insisted that "man is φύσει πολιτικός, [and] that apart from the community he is θεός ἢ θήριον, no man at all".[6] Hobbes, by contrast, links solitariness to existence in a state of nature, but takes the state of nature to be unremittingly awful[7]; the upshot is that, once again, sociality is preferable to asociality. Sentiments such as this may be interpreted as reflecting an attitude along the lines that being let alone may be desirable from time to time, but should not be seen as an unqualified good: even if being let alone occasionally is a *part* of flourishing, that is not the part that was emphasised. Warren and Brandeis reverse this, emphasising the importance of separateness from others as essential for wellbeing; and a right to privacy accordingly protects against intrusions into agents' mental and social lives in much the same way that rights of bodily integrity protect against intrusions into their lives *qua* physical beings. It is striking that Warren and Brandeis characterise violations of privacy as being more distressing than "mere bodily injury".

Yet what a right to be let alone would mean for genetic privacy is not straightforward. On the face of things, the applicability of the RLA account seems reasonably clear: if privacy is a matter of being able to separate oneself from others, and to withdraw to some extent from the unwanted attention of others, then being able to withdraw genetic information, or ensure its not being disseminated, ought to be of a piece with that. And yet this presupposes that there is a significant overlap between the violation of privacy represented by the paparazzo pointing his camera through the starlet's window, and the putative violation of privacy we see in a case like Gerry and Terry's. There may not be.

This is because information about what starlets get up to behind closed doors is, *per* the terminology I introduced in chapter 1, confined. It sounds pleonastic, but to find out what the starlet does behind closed doors, one has to find out what she does behind closed doors. Genetic information is not like that. In order to find out at least some things about the people with whom one shares a genome, one only has to find out about oneself. In this way, Gerry isn't really doing anything with or to Terry when he finds out information about himself that will reveal his identical twin brother's genome to him. Terry doesn't need to be visible to Gerry, or touchable, or even on the same continent. Crucially, Gerry is not not-letting-Terry-alone, or encroaching upon his person, by any normal understanding of the term (and certainly not by Warren and Brandeis's). And so, if the RLA account is correct, the idea that Gerry is doing something to his brother that would violate his privacy is a little hard to accept, at least without further argument. Correlatively, the right to be let alone would seem on its most natural reading to mean *people* being let alone. But genetic information is not people; it is information *about* people. It is people, not information, that are supposed to have rights. And while one may bother people in the process of learning information about them, it is presumably possible not to: as noted a moment ago, we can obtain information about a blood relative's genome without being remotely close to them. And so it would follow that, if the RLA account is correct, Terry's right to privacy is not violated after all when Gerry finds out something about his genome.

Taken together, this would amount to saying that genetic privacy turns out to be no such thing: if a right to privacy is a right to be let alone, and if a right to be let alone does not engage with genetics, then there is no right to genetic privacy. Conversely, if we want to say that there is such a thing as genetic privacy (and that it is something to which someone might have a right) it is not obvious that the RLA account can give us what we need – unless we think that Gerry fails to let his brother alone by finding out about his own genome, which I think implausible. If we want to maintain a right to genetic privacy, we would have to look beyond the RLA account. This ought not to be catastrophic if it is true that other accounts of the right to privacy are developments of or derivatives from it: the very need for developments implies as much.

There is a further shortcoming in the RLA account that does not depend on its having generated problems for Terry's privacy claim; this is that, as Charles Fried suggests, it would appear imply that Robinson Crusoe has perfect privacy. After all, a man on a desert island is let alone entirely. Yet it would seem to be more natural simply to say that he was entirely deprived of company than that he enjoyed perfect privacy.[8] It does not take a great deal to see what the problem here is: to have a *right* to privacy implies waivability, and the ability to take others into our confidence. Equally, it implies the ability not to require others to leave us alone. Robinson Crusoe can waive his right to privacy in only the most notional of ways. If a right to privacy is just a matter of a right to be let alone, it is not a right that Crusoe enjoys after all, since it is not something he can relinquish. And so it would appear that privacy, at least as the word is normally used, is *not* (or is not entirely) a matter of being let alone, nor of information about a person remaining un-accessed by others, and that a right to privacy is *not* simply a matter of a right to be let alone. We have a reason, therefore, to modify the RLA account at the very least.

It is interesting to note, finally, that there may be ways in which asserting a right to be let alone could militate *against* genetic privacy for at least some people. This is a possibility raised by a point made by Bayevsky and Berkman in respect of pre-natal genetic testing,[9] though it is not one that they develop. Allow that among an agent's reproductive rights are rights to be allowed to manage reproduction as they see fit, without outside interference by other agents (including, but not limited to, the state). Thus people would be able to access contraception, women would be able to access abortion, and so on. This negative reproductive liberty right is clearly coeval with privacy *qua* right to be let alone. Now: the right to make reproductive decisions, Bayevsky and Berkman argue, implies a right to information about the genome of the foetus. Immediately, this would mean that no right to privacy could be asserted on behalf of the foetus, or of the child-to-be: it is not wronged by some other person having come to know the details of its genome even before it was aware of itself. (The claim that the foetus has no privacy rights ought not to be all that big a surprise, of course, since it is perfectly conventional to insist that a foetus has no rights to begin with, and that neither does a merely future person.) But if the mother's right to make reproductive decisions implies a right to information about the genome of the foetus, it looks as though the father's privacy may be eroded as well, even though he definitely is a person and definitely does exist in the present. After all, a mother who learned something about her child's genome as a part of making her own reproductive decisions would thereby likely gain an insight into the father's genome, even if it is only probabilistic. For example, in discovering that the foetus carried the Huntington gene, she would know that there is a 50% chance that it came from the father; and knowing something about his family history would give her a more significant insight into his genome even without his having had a genetic test.

In other words, if reproductive rights imply a right to access information about the foetus, it looks as though fathers will not have these privacy rights, because at least one person would appear to have access to information about his genome as a matter of *her* right. And if (as Bayevsky and Berkman suggest) American jurisprudence is correct to link reproductive rights to privacy rights, then it looks – paradoxically – as though the father's privacy rights are eroded by the mother's.[10] Of course, the way out of this paradox is to point out that if a right to privacy is a right to be let alone, it does not follow that all rights to be let alone are privacy rights: whatever their similarities, there could be a distinction to be drawn between rights to be let alone *qua* privacy, and rights to be let alone *qua* negative liberty. Even so, if a woman's reproductive liberty really does imply a right to access genetic information about the foetus she is carrying, then the father's right to genetic privacy is moot. And if privacy is a matter of being let alone, then it is not obvious that the father would be able to appeal to it to prevent access to his genome anyway, because – as we have just seen – it is not obvious that the RLA account is up to the job. He would not be inconvenienced by his genetic information being known to the mother: he would not be not-let-alone.

The long and the short of it is that, if there is a right to genetic privacy, it is not best understood as a right to be let alone. Perhaps, though, there is more to privacy than a right to be let alone. As we shall see over the coming pages, it may be possible to conceptualise it as a matter of control of access to the self.

(b) Privacy as Control over Access to Self

A slightly more sophisticated account of the putative right to privacy pivots from a concern about being let alone, to a concern about being able to control and limit access to the self. Call this the Access-to-Self, or AtS, account. Privacy, as explained by Richard Parker in his rehearsal of the AtS account, "is control over when and by whom the (physical) parts of us (as identifiable persons) can be seen or heard (in person or by use of photographs, recordings, TV, etc.), touched, smelled, or tasted by others".[11] This account offers less of a way to answer the Robinson Crusoe objection than a way not to have to address it, since there is no access that needs controlling; and it seems to explain what has been violated in the example of the paparazzo and the starlet, since she has lost control of the sensory access that others have to her.

An important characteristic of the account is the role played by identifiability. If information about a person cannot be linked to them, then their self remains inaccessible, and so there would be no breach of privacy or any right to privacy. And so it is that, at least as Parker presents the AtS account, while it may seem that one person reading another's diary would be a paradigmatic case of privacy violation, we may have to be a bit more circumspect. Equally, we can lose control over private information (whether that was because we shared it or because we were careless with it) without necessarily losing privacy; as such, "[i]f we tell someone that we are homosexual, we lose control over private information, but we do not necessarily lose privacy".[12] Information *about* a self can be divorced from that self, and for private information to be de-privatised does not necessarily affect the privacy of the self to which it refers. Hence

> a single line in a diary might identify to the onlooker the identity of the author of the diary and greatly increase his loss of control over who could sense part of him; [but i]f he remains anonymous, he retains control over who can sense him as a distinct individual.[13]

If privacy is lost, then the content of the diary will determine the severity of that loss, but nothing more; but the *if* clause has to be satisfied. It is not the content of the diary that determines whether privacy has been lost to begin with; and "the information revealed when we are sensed does not affect the degree of the loss in privacy, *i.e.*, the loss of control over when and by whom we are sensed".[14] Ruth Gavison has an appreciably similar account; for her, privacy is at least in some sense a matter of accessibility, and privacy may be undermined when we seek out information about identifiable others.[15]

The relevance of this for genetic information ought to be clear. If someone accesses information about my genome, I would not necessarily have had my privacy rights violated, provided that that information was anonymised. Johnson *et al*'s claim that we ought to be willing to share our genetic information for the sake of the public good, but that stringent data protection policies should be put in place to guarantee privacy,[16] makes most sense when seen through this kind of lens: information could be reasonably freely shared without privacy rights being put at risk so long as the chance of identifiability was nugatory at most. On the other hand, since Gerry will know that information about himself is also information about his twin, Terry's privacy will be violated when Gerry learns about his own genome – and the principle applies in a modified form in respect of other blood relatives. That would seem to indicate that, if the AtS is the correct account, there can be no thoroughgoing right to genetic privacy within a familial context, since all information about oneself will reveal information about identifiable others, giving each of us access to blood relatives' selves; and protecting those selves would diminish our ability to access our *own* selves – which is, *per* the argument of chapter 2, inimical to the idea of privacy properly understood.

Although I am making use of Parker's account mainly for illustrative purposes, it's still worth noting a few perplexities that it raises. In respect of the example of telling someone about one's homosexuality, I think it would be perfectly natural to want to say that privacy *was* diminished, insofar as that it was wittingly surrendered. In telling someone about our sexuality, what are we doing if *not* providing them with access to at least an aspect of our self – access of which they were hitherto in a state of privation? (This is compatible with the speaker taking the listener into his confidence, or telling him a secret.) But more important is the objection that saying that non-identifiability implies no violation of loss of privacy rights does not seem quite correct. Suppose that someone finds a diary and makes himself comfortable in order to have a good read. In that case, it seems natural to want to say that he has violated privacy rights in some sense from the moment he opens the covers, before even there's been a chance for any identifying information to be disclosed.

Yet there could be a response to this, built around a modified account of the self that is being accessed. Perhaps we could and should treat something like a diary as an aspect of the "extended self". A diary is something into which we consciously make some kind of existential investment, and having it read by others without our permission *is* after all, we might want to say, a case of our having ceded control over access to our self. We talk about a writer pouring himself into his diary; well, in that case, accessing the diary means accessing the poured component of the self. Reading the diary does not just give the reader access to information *about* the diarist, but access in a real sense to a *part of* the diarist. The need for identifiability would be diminished by this move, since someone could have access to an extended self without having to tie it to a particular person. Likewise, the paparazzo with his camera trained on the starlet's house intrudes into her extended self in some meaningful way, even if all he does is to take photos of her décor. Indeed, that might help us explain why a right to be let alone might have struck us as important: it has a kind of existential aspect, not a million miles away from what Sartre called "being-for-others".[17] For sure, there will likely always be a part of the extended self that is irreducibly public, such that perfect privacy could be maintained only by withdrawing from public life. But even if some of the extended self is public, not all of it must be. What one writes in a diary is the sort of thing that one might perfectly reasonably expect to remain outside of the public or interpersonal domains, short of some positive intervention to make it accessible. And so it may be that access to the (extended) self *is* available when information that is in some sense *about* the self becomes accessible to others. Thinking in this way has the added advantage of keeping the AtS account true to its own nature, by saving it from collapsing into a control-of-information account, which is subtly different, and which I shall consider in a moment.

That said, it is still not clear how that argument would give us quite what we want when it comes to genetic privacy, and much of the reason for this is because of genetic information's unconfinement. Even if we want to say that genetic information does give access to the self, extended or otherwise, it is not about *only* the self – it is about others' selves, too. In one sense, even the extended self version of the argument doesn't go far enough here. Suppose we voluntarily share genetic information about ourselves: in doing so, we are granting access to our (extended) selves, but also to that of others. If that is to violate a right held by those others, it implies that we have at least a *prima facie* reason not to allow third parties access to our genomes; but this makes privacy no longer a right but a duty. More, in discovering about our own genome, we would be discovering about others', and so accessing their extended self; were that to violate a right of theirs – as Terry found in the last chapter – we would risk self-knowledge becoming forbidden.

Moreover, while appeals to an extended self may help explain the sense of a violation of privacy rights in respect of things like diaries or photographs, it is not at all clear that genetics would fit the model in the same way, because individuals do not identify themselves by their genes – or, at least, genes are a long way down the league-table of important ways in which people identify themselves. If Alice learns about Bob's genome, it is really not his self or the integrity of that self that is violated in the same way. What has been violated, though, is his ability to control information about himself. And so it is that it would appear that, fairly quickly, we have to shift from an Access-to-Self account, to a Control over Personal Information account in order to make sense of genetic privacy.

There is one final objection to an AtS account that is worth making, though, not least because it will resonate later; this is that it comes "too late". Suppose that genetic information is anonymised, such that the person accessing it will never have any sense of the referent. And allow that – as I suspect may be true – nobody identifies with their genomes in the way that they identify with their diaries. If the AtS account is right, this ought to soothe our concerns about access to genetic information. But I do not think that our concerns would be soothed. This is because someone who embarks on the quest for information about others is engaged in the process of wrenching information into "his" realm: information of which he had previously been deprived. The reader of the diary may not know, and may never know, whose diary he is reading – but he has still wrested information into a realm where it was not previously. More, he has engaged in attempting to wrest it into the interpersonal realm even if those attempts fail - say because the diary is written in a code or a foreign language. It seems natural to say that this is a wrong. Similarly, the paparazzo has acted wrongly from the moment he points his lens through the starlet's window, irrespective of what information, if any, he will go on to glean, and irrespective even of whether he knows or cares whose house he is looking at. The best explanation for this sense of wrong is that privacy rights have been violated.

Of course, there are other candidate explanations. One would be that the wrong is not best explained as a violation of any of the starlet's or the diarist's privacy rights so long as they remained unidentifiable; rather, the wrong lies in the creation of a *chance* of identification: that privacy is put at risk, and that there is a wrong to putting privacy at risk that is not quite the same as violating privacy itself. I might feel aggrieved if some action of yours makes it more likely that I will be identifiable as the referent of some piece of information. But that grievance may be warranted on its own terms; the violation of privacy about which I am worried would be a matter for further complaint.

Yet this does not seem entirely convincing. For one thing, it seems to amount to reasserting the disputed formulation; we probably would want to say that our privacy, and our right to privacy, had been violated even if nothing that identified us came to light. But the nub of the "too-late" objection is that, if I am right to say that the essence of the private is that information is not in the interpersonal domain, then a right to privacy would seem to be inseparable from a right not to have it brought into that domain, and being identifiable does not obviously have much to do with that. My privacy right, if there is one, is a right that you not snuffle information out. Your being able to tie snuffled-out information to me may mean that I am harmed in a way that I would not be were unidentifiability preserved; but the right does not depend on that. As Stanley Benn puts matters,

> it is not that [things] are kept out of sight or from the knowledge of others that makes them private. Rather, they are matters that it would be inappropriate for others to try to find out about, much less report on, without one's consent; one complains if they are publicized precisely because they are private. Similarly, a private room remains private in spite of uninvited intruders, for falsifying the expectation that no one will intrude is not a logically sufficient ground for saying that something private in this sense is not private after all.[18]

To complain about a violation of privacy rights is not to complain that someone can identify us; it is to complain that they have tried to wrest control of relevant information from us full stop.

(c) Privacy as Control over Personal Information

It is not beyond the realms of possibility that there could be ways to make an Access-to-Self account of privacy accommodate claims about control of information – say, by treating (control over) access to information as (control over) access to some version of an extended self. But it may be difficult to shake the suspicion that such accommodation is a little grudging. It is much more efficient to admit that privacy really is simply about control of access to personal information.

It was Charles Fried who dismissed the RLA account by raising the point that, by its lights, Robinson Crusoe does not enjoy privacy; and his counterposition is articulated in the claim that the essence of privacy and privacy rights lies in our ability to control *information* about ourselves:

As a first approximation, privacy seems to be related to secrecy, to limiting the knowledge of others about oneself. This notion must be refined. It is not true, for instance, that the less that is known about us the more privacy we have. Privacy is not simply an absence of information about us in the minds of others; rather it is the *control* we have over information about ourselves.[19]

Elsewhere, he states that privacy is "control over knowledge about oneself",[20] and that it is "that aspect of social order by which persons control access to information about themselves. [… I]t is a feeling of security in control over that information".[21] Fried's definition of privacy is a little different from the idea I outlined in chapter 2; but insofar as that either way a right to privacy would involve being able to stop others bringing information into the interpersonal domain, this does not matter all that much. It also looks promising if we want to provide an account of how Terry's privacy might have been violated by Gerry's having had a genetic test. A Control-over-Personal-Information (CoPI) account is clearly not a million miles away from the AtS account (and I think that it is fair to say that Gavison's account has characteristics of both), but it does make explicit reference to information. It is on this basis that I shall include Anita Allen's account in the group of CoPI theories of privacy, since she offers a definition of privacy that denotes "inaccessibility of persons, of their mental states, *and of information about them* to the senses and surveillance devices of others".[22] And while Solove complains that the CoPI account is probably too narrow to provide a full account of privacy – "it excludes those aspects of privacy that are not informational, such as the right to make certain fundamental decisions about one's body, reproduction, or rearing of one's children"[23] – this does not concern me too much here: informational privacy is my focus.

A good recent outing of an account that clearly belongs in the CoPI family can be found in Andrei Marmor's 2015 paper on the right to privacy, which posits that a right to privacy is best understood as deriving from a general interest that people have in being able to control the way in which they present themselves to others, at least within reasonable limits.[24] Information is a major part of that position, such that "a violation of a right to privacy is not simply about *what is known* but mostly about the ways in which some *information* is obtained".[25] Our ability to control the way in which we are presented to others is, he contends, a crucial part of our wellbeing; a right to privacy is properly understood as being the right that safeguards that, and ensures that the terms on which we relate to others are reasonably predictable. While some other parties might have a legitimate interest in certain pieces of information about us, and that interest may suffice to mean that we ought to surrender that information to them, the fact that we might on occasion be expected to provide information to some people does not imply that we have to be entirely candid to all people all the time. Thus though we would normally regard information about our finances as private, it does not follow that we may withhold them from the tax authorities; but the fact that we should provide that information to the authorities does not mean that we have to provide them to everyone that asks – or even, really, that the tax authorities themselves have a free pass to access information about our finances. (This line of argument will prove to be very useful for the position I shall outline in the final two chapters of this book.)

One of the attractions of an account like Marmor's is that it is better than Fried's at biting into the Gerry and Terry problem. Fried builds into his account of the importance of privacy familiar concerns for political liberty and so on, but emphasises that "privacy is the necessary context for relationships which we would hardly be human if we had to do without – the relationships of love, friendship and trust".[26] The support that privacy gives to important human relationships is perhaps the single most important theme in his account. But it is not clear what this would mean for people in a situation like Gerry and Terry's. Fried is concerned to show that privacy is "not just a defensive right" – a right to keep others out of our lives – but that it is a necessary part of love and friendship, insofar as that it ensures the exclusive nature of particular states of love and trust.[27] But that kind of relationship is not what is at stake in the Gerry and Terry problem. They are not intimates, the special nature of whose relationship is guaranteed by the rights and privileges of privacy, and so the thing that makes Fried's account provocative and interesting is inapplicable here. Equally, if expectations of trust and intimacy are what *motivate* concerns about privacy, it looks as though privacy may have little to contribute to understanding any dispute between close relatives about access to genetic information, since privacy in this case is not so much protecting a bond of trust and intimacy as it is marking the line of control between two disputing parties. Note that Fried does not say that privacy is not a defensive right at all: only that it is not *just* one – but having decided that his appeals to love and friendship do not apply here indicates that we would likely have to retreat to the defensive aspect of privacy. As such, Fried's account is worth noting, but would not be something upon which Terry could build a case before any hypothetical tribunal.

Other accounts of privacy appeal to the importance of control of information, and so clearly belong in the CoPI family, emphasising not so much the way that information is shared in the first place, as what is done with it once it has been shared. Thus, for Wright Clayton *et al*,

> [t]he traditional view of privacy as secrecy or concealment – as a 'right to be let alone' – has grown increasingly strained in the Information Age. [...] A new theorization of privacy has emerged, in which concealing one's secrets 'is less relevant than being in control of the distribution and use by others' of the data people generate in the course of seeking healthcare, conducting consumer transactions, and going about their lives.[28]

Accordingly, the analysis of the law that they offer is informed by the idea that respecting and maintaining privacy is a matter of guaranteeing, and perhaps increasing, individuals' control over disclosures by others that may affect them.[29] Such an account seems to sit reasonably straightforwardly with Marmor's. But while this account casts a useful light on the question of privacy – and one that will be relevant later – I do not think that it would help with the Gerry and Terry problem, the nub of which is not to do with what Gerry may do with the information once he's got it, as it is to do with whether or not he may get it in the first place. I shall, therefore, take Marmor as providing my example of what a CoPI account would look like.

Marmor acknowledges that there are certain kinds of information that we cannot hope to control and that therefore cannot come under the purview of a right to privacy. I cannot claim that people violate my privacy rights by noticing that I am walking along the street. We differentiate between others learning things about me in such a way as to violate my privacy, and their learning things about me in such a way as not to, by means of an appeal to what we can control. Thus

> your right to privacy is violated when somebody manipulates, without adequate justification, the relevant environment in ways that significantly diminish your ability to control what aspects of yourself you reveal to others.[30]

The idea of adequate justification, and the question of what might count as adequate, are matters to which I'll return in chapters 6 to 8. For the time being, we should simply note that Marmor is saying that the essence of the violation of a privacy right lies in others having manipulated the environment in order to make information more accessible than it would otherwise be.[31]

This is considerably more satisfying than an AtS account, and it fits nicely with the definition of the private I offered in chapter 2, which treats it as that which is by default not on public view – that for which someone has to go looking. Equally, we can infer that privacy can be shed without there being a violation. For example, someone might undress and go for a swim on a hot day, believing that they are in a secluded cove, but not realising that they can easily be seen from the path along the cliff; though the swimmer may thereby be showing more than they intend (and might be embarrassed to learn the truth of the matter), we would not want to say that their being seen would necessarily indicate a violation of privacy, because there is no manipulation of the relevant environment (or if there is, it is by the swimmer: nobody ese is implicated). Along similar lines, we might imagine cases of what one might call "farcical misfortune", as when curtain-rails collapse at inopportune moments, the wind blows loose clothing awry, and so on. Any privacy right that we have in such situations is likely to be – to borrow Rumbold and Wilson's term – defunct.[32] A defunct right would be a right that it is impossible for anyone to satisfy or that generates duties that it is impossible for any putative duty-bearer to discharge. Things would have been brought into the public or interpersonal domain, but, since nobody would have manipulated the environment, we would want to say that there had been at most a *loss*, rather than a *violation*. (Marmor hints that there might be situations in which one might waive privacy rights, too – these would be situations in which one is doing something in public that belongs in the private realm; but here, it's not really privacy that's in play, so much as the integrity of the public realm.[33])

That said, Marmor does think that privacy brings with it certain duties in the event that it is unwittingly breached:

> When you take a walk on Main Street, you are perfectly aware of the fact that you have no control over who happens to be there and thus is able to see you; but you also rely on the fact that people's attention and memory are very limited. You do not expect to have every tiny movement of yours noticed and recorded by others. In other words, consent to public exposure is not unlimited. Voluntarily giving indefinite others the opportunity to see you is not an invitation, or even tacit consent, to gaze at you, and certainly not a consent to record your doings, digitally or otherwise.[34]

Correspondingly, Rumbold and Wilson point out that there may be privacy-related rights and duties that are not rendered defunct by circumstance. In a farcical misfortune situation, one's right not to be *seen* in a particular way is defunct; but there would still be a right not be *looked at* that is not quite the same, and a right that witnesses not say too much about what they have seen. Again, this fits with my claim in chapter 2 about privacy implying a duty to let go, mentally, of things that one has come to know when one ought not to have come to know them. It also fits with what I shall have to say later about prying.

Marmor's account of privacy rights as enabling control over access to personal information is attractive. Still, I am not sure that, *qua* right, it would quite give us what we need when trying to get to grips with genetic information, and with Gerry's putative violation of Terry's privacy; and my concerns with Marmor's account are indicative of the kinds of concern that we might have with CoPI accounts across the board.

One question that presents itself concerns what it means to talk about manipulating the environment; and, correspondingly, any CoPI account must be able to say what it is to wrest control of information. One sense of the word "manipulate" implies instrumentality: Alice would violate Bob's privacy by setting out to arrange affairs in such a way as to mean that she will discover something about Bob that she might otherwise not have discovered. Call this "hard manipulation". On this account, hacking emails or (less plausibly) making use of x-ray goggles deliberately to look into someone's house would violate privacy rights. Marmor, however, wants the word "manipulate" to be understood in a softer sense, which would extend to cover cases in which one discovered facts about another inadvertently. If someone sees inside his neighbour's safe while testing his x-ray goggles, there will have been a violation of privacy (though whether it is a *wrongful* violation would be a further question).[35] Soft manipulation may still have to arise from a deliberate act: the goggle-user is deliberately using the goggles, although this particular outcome of their use was unintended. A violation of putative genetic privacy may arise from hard manipulation: one person may set out specifically to discover information about another's genome, and arrange affairs in such a way as to facilitate that; but it is also entirely possible that it is from soft manipulation. This would cover cases in which one discovers information about another person as a side-effect of finding out about oneself. Nobody takes a genetic test by accident; but in the excitement of finding out something about himself, it might never have occurred to an agent that the genetic privacy of family members is at stake. Yet the agent in this scenario has still (on Marmor's account) manipulated the environment in such a way as to mean that blood relatives lose at least some control over the way information about them is revealed to at least one other person.

But is this really how we would want to describe matters? It is not obvious that by taking the genetic test anyone has manipulated the environment in any particularly meaningful, or at least relevant, way, be it hard or soft. As we saw a moment ago, merely becoming aware of something that would normally be considered private does not imply that the person who becomes aware of it has manipulated affairs in such a way as to reduce referents' control of information. The walker strolling along the headland who happens to notice the naked swimmer has not manipulated the environment – certainly not so as to learn something about that swimmer. By analogy, we may want to be careful about saying that the person who has a genetic test has manipulated the environment so as to learn about blood relatives. What may be true is that any responsible agent should be aware of the fact that, in learning about himself, he will also learn something about others, and should take that into account. But it is not clear how far we would want to take this line, for fear of committing ourselves to the absurd idea that it may be wrong to walk along the headland just in case one sees others removing their clothes for what they think is a secluded swim.[36] And if being negligent of the possible consequences of an action is a wrong, it is not one that relies on any right having been violated.[37]

Perhaps more importantly, if we try to apply the CoPI account to a case like Gerry and Terry's, we will see that there is a huge problem for it. Terry's privacy would rely on his having control over his information; but (as we saw in the last chapter) that would seem to imply that Gerry would have a duty to remain in ignorance of his own genome – and thereby undermine his control over personal information. And since control over personal information was what privacy rights are supposed to protect, then those privacy rights themselves look to be imperilled.[38] As argued in the last chapter, the twins' genomes would have moved from the realm of the private into the realm of the secret or the taboo. In Kantian terms, Terry's maxim of controlling personal information could not be universalised, and so could not really be used to generate rights or duties.

There is another difficulty. What counts as manipulation to begin with? Imagine that Bob and Mary are both given a safe, each of which requires a different combination to open. Each is told that combination, told that they may look into their own safe, and that they are under no obligation to tell the combination to each other. Imagine too that each safe has identical or near-identical contents, and Bob and Mary both know this. Suppose Bob opens his safe. For sure, he has manipulated the environment; and in doing so he has learned something about the content of Mary's safe. But it would be strange to think that he had violated Mary's privacy; neither would we want to say that Bob had manipulated the environment in the right sort of way to make that a worry – in fact, *her* environment does not seem to have been manipulated at all. By parity of reasoning, we might wonder what Gerry has done to manipulate Terry's environment by doing the genetic equivalent of looking in his own safe. What, then, is the relevant environment? Just as Bob is not doing anything to Mary or anything that Mary owns, neither would Gerry be doing anything to Terry or to anything that Terry owns, at least inasmuch as that the blood test, or swab, or whatever, would come from Gerry's body rather than Terry's; and the information would not be "owned" by Terry – not exclusively, anyway.

iii. Privacy and Property

At this point, I would like to linger for a moment to the idea that we see in Marmor's account that information is at least in some relevant way similar to private property. This similarity works in one of two ways. In one, information is something that one might treat as being like property in its own right, and it can be treated in the same sort of way – as something that can be bought, sold, appropriated, misappropriated, and so on. So, then, when considering the wrong that is done to a person whose phone calls have been logged by a party other than the phone company, he claims that a privacy right is violated, and that

> it seems that the right that [the person who logged your calls] violated has something to do with the fact that he obtained something that is essentially yours, without your permission. Perhaps the list of your calls is not quite your property, but it is close enough.[39]

Information has been obtained in something like the way that a thing might be obtained, and rights over private information might be violated in roughly the way that rights over private property could be violated.

Left like this, the objection to this analogy is that information is unlike medium-sized solid objects in at least one important way: whereas my having obtained something from you generally means that you have less of it, that is not true of information. If I violate your property rights by stealing your bag of humbugs, you have fewer humbugs to enjoy. But information, when mis-appropriated, is more often copied than moved – so whether it really is like enough to one's physical property (and whether it is "essentially yours" in the way that medium-sized solid objects might be) is not by any means a settled matter.

The other way the analogy works is a little more indirect, inasmuch as that information itself need not be something owned; but it is important because of what it tells us about the things that one *does* own. If Bob learns through the use of his x-ray goggles that Mary has in her safe either an unflattering nude portrait of her husband, or, in another scenario, a Picasso – either way, something that she would prefer be kept from prying eyes – then he has vio-lated her privacy. But this would not be because the information *is* private property in its own right, but because it *refers to* private property. Bob "manipulates the environment in ways that undermine Mary's ability to con-trol how she presents herself or, actually, *what is hers* to others",[40] and this is the violation of her privacy, and so of any privacy right that may be in play. This approach does seem not to be vulnerable to the copying objection voiced a moment ago: symbolically at least, Bob would have wrested from Mary something to which she had previously thought she had exclusive access.

What unites these two ways of thinking about information – be it private information proper, or information about private property – is that we can use the language of ownership. Information about my telephone calls is "mine", because it relates to things that are proper to me. There might be circumstances in which other parties have a legal and even a moral right to wrest this information from me; but these would be departures from the default situation in which I can choose who, if anyone, should have access to it. Mary can say that information about whether or not she has a Picasso in her safe is "hers" – she is the arbiter of who gets that information; medical information, in a similar sort of way, is mine. All of this suggests that ownership of information is compatible with privacy talk in something like the way that ownership of medium-sized solid objects is compatible with privacy talk. If this kind of thought has heft to it, it might be taken as an indication that it could be brought to bear to questions about how to deal with genetic information.

But it is not after all easy to see how well the analogy works in respect of genetic information. For one thing, information about the contents of Mary's safe is information about the things that Mary does or does not own. Information about genes or genomes may not be analogous, because it is not clear that genes and genomes are things that one might own in the sense of having exclusive title. Colloquially, of course, we might talk about "your" or "my" genes or genome; but we ought to be a little wary of reading too much into these figures of speech.

One reason to be suspicious of the analogy is that it is a key feature of most property that one can alienate – that is to say, get rid of – it. But one cannot alienate one's genes: one cannot separate oneself from them in a way that one can separate oneself from a Picasso. Granted, genes are not genetic information; so the impossibility of alienating genes tells us little about the possibility of alienating information about them. Although one cannot give information away and so alienate it in precisely the way that one can alienate an object – this is the copying objection again – there are other ways in which one perhaps may alienate information fairly easily. For example, if one gives away or burns the piece of paper on which information about a genome is written, then this looks like it is alienating information; one's memory of what was written on that paper would also fade, which is another kind of alienation. (Information has a half-life – a rate of natural erosion – that makes it liable slowly to disappear from one's "ownership" unless it is preserved in what I have called elsewhere the "external archive".[41]) One might possess things without knowing it, too; and information may sometimes be thought of in those terms. Presumably, were you to surreptitiously run a cholesterol test on me, I might say that you had violated my privacy, and mean by it that you had got access to what is mine or relates directly to what is mine.

All the same, and granted that we are happy enough to admit that *some* information can be in some sense "mine" (or be closely tied to things like paintings that are mine), it doesn't follow that all can. The basic point stands that there is a plausible difference between genetic and other kinds of information that should be fairly clear based on the distinction between confined and unconfined information that I introduced earlier. Genetic information is unconfined, and it is not obvious how the possessive pronoun might work in that context. For sure, a third party's running a genetic test on me looks to be at least something like their running a cholesterol test, and so I might want to say that there is a right against third parties that does not hold against blood relatives; but the standard model of bioethics has it that my right to privacy is blind to who is seeking information. At the very least, more would have to be said; and the more qualifications and nuances we add to the story, the less robust the putative right looks. As I shall argue later, it may be more simple just to abandon the idea that the right is a *datum* in debates about who ought to have access to what.

The nub of the problem in the Gerry and Terry example is precisely that the information belongs exclusively to neither, and is exclusively about neither; and although the congruence between two given individuals' genomes will fade the less closely they are related, there will still be some significant degree of "shared tenure" among blood relatives. There will be an echo of this point when we consider the "joint account" model of genetic information a little later. Mary can claim that the picture in the safe is hers, and that information about that picture is closely tied to what is hers, because information about her art collection is not information about others' art collections – save in the very etiolated sense that our knowing that Mary has exclusive title over a painting tells us that nobody else owns it. Likewise, the owner of a phone can say that the list of calls is a way of presenting information that is his, inasmuch as that he is the ultimate referent, and he can exclude others from accessing it. Finally, a person can often talk about medical information in this sense, because (say) their kidney or their body wholesale is *theirs*: granted that the body cannot be alienated, one can still distinguish between one's own and other people's bodies, or those other bodies themselves. Terry cannot easily make any similar claim, because (to return to the telephone analogy) Gerry's and Terry's genomes are less like different telephone lines than they are like the upstairs and downstairs handsets of a household landline. And this spells trouble for the information-as-property model if we try to apply it too quickly to genetic information: the presuppositions that underpin the ownership of, and privacy rights over, the former do not translate to the latter.

And, of course, even if we grant that privacy is a matter of control over information, we have already seen that this implies being able to access information about oneself. Hence Terry's privacy claims would engage Gerry's directly, and not just by way of appeals to informational privilege. Yet this brings us right back to the problem. Terry's protecting his putative privacy is therefore less like Mary hiding her painting away from prying eyes than it is like her intercepting Bob's post to make sure he never gets his x-ray goggles.

And so, if we're to make sense of Terry's putative privacy rights, a model such as Marmor's, in which privacy is the thing violated when the control that an agent has over the way in which she presents herself to the world is diminished through another's manipulation of the environment, does not sit easily when it comes to genetics. Or, to put it another way, if Marmor is right, it is not immediately obvious that we can make sense of the idea that Terry's privacy rights are violated by Gerry learning about his and their genome after all.

iv. Stepping Back

A brief recap may be in order.

An invasion of privacy, and the concomitant violation of a right to privacy, may be understood as a loss of a right to be let alone, or as a loss of control over access to the self, or as a loss of control over personal information, or as the loss of control over property: all would be erosions of this privilege. The problem is that none of these accounts seems to be all that well-fitted to helping us think clearly about genetic privacy and conflicts concerning it. None of them really provides a satisfactory way to think about something like genetic information. Privacy understood as a right to be let alone does not seem to fit when Terry is not particularly inconvenienced by his brother's having a genetic test; and if control over personal information can be said to be at stake, this cuts both ways: one brother's maintaining control over information involves the other's losing it. By placing less emphasis on control, access-to-self accounts sidestep this problem; but the price paid is that it is neither clear that access to genetic information is access to the self in the right sort of way, or that an agent can prevent blood relatives' access to his self as a matter of right without at the same time limiting their access to their own selves, thereby nudging genetic information from the realm of the private into the realm of the taboo. Finally, while control of personal information accounts may offer a promising way to think about privacy rights, they do not seem to apply so easily to genetic information, which imperils the idea that there is a right in play at all.

This chapter has focused on the main theoretical accounts of what a privacy right might be. In the next chapter, I shall consider Graeme Laurie's account of privacy rights, which is notably different (and has different concerns) from the theories considered here; I shall also look at reasons for a kind of reductionism about privacy rights – and I shall conclude that neither of these will help us keep hold of all the facets of informational privilege when it comes to our genomes. However, it is possible that there is another account, not considered here, that would be able to give us a way to explain putative rights to genetic privacy. In chapter 6, I shall turn my attention to practical concerns, and argue that *even if* there is a model that could provide a clear understanding of genetic privacy claims in theory, there are likely still to be moral barriers to applying it in practice.

Notes

1 Solove, D, "Conceptualizing Privacy", *California Law Review* 90[4] (2002): 1087–1156; *Understanding Privacy* (Cambridge, Mass: Harvard UP, 2009), *passim*.
2 Warren, S, & Brandeis, L, "The Right to Privacy", *Harvard Law Review* 4[5] (1890), pp 195–196.
3 *ibid*, p 196.
4 *Roe v Wade*, 410 U.S. 113 (1973), at 168.
5 Aristotle, *The Politics* (London: Penguin, 1992), 1253a1.
6 Bradley, FH, *Ethical Studies* (London: HS King, 1976), p 171.
7 Hobbes, T, *Leviathan* (Cambridge: Cambridge UP, 1999), p 89.
8 Fried, C, "Privacy", *Yale Law Journal* 77[3] (1968), p 482.
9 Bayefsky, M, & Berkman, B, "Implementing Expanded Prenatal Genetic Testing: Should Parents Have Access to Any and All Fetal Genetic Information?" *The American Journal of Bioethics*, 22[2] (2022), p 12.
10 An important interjection must be made here: Justice Alito's opinion in the US Supreme Court's judgment in the case of *Dobbs v Jackson Women's Health Organisation* (597 U.S. ___ (2022)) denies that the attempt in *Roe v Wade* to ground abortion rights in privacy rights succeeded; this is on the basis that there is no Constitutional right to privacy to begin with. However, rights that Constitutional law may or may not grant do not necessarily speak to moral rights that we may have.
11 Parker, R, "A Definition of Privacy", *Rutgers Law Review* 27[2] (1974), pp 283–284.
12 *ibid*, p 282 (slightly modified).
13 *ibid*, p 283.
14 *ibid*, p 283.

15 Gavison, R, "Privacy and the Limits of Law", *Yale Law Journal* 89[3] (1980), p 434.

16 Johnson, S *et al*, "Rethinking the Ethical Principles of Genomic Medicine Services", *European Journal of Human Genetics* 28 (2020), *passim*.

17 Sartre, J-P, *Being and Nothingness* (London: Routledge, 1995), *passim*.

18 Benn, S, "Privacy, Freedom, and Respect for Persons", in Schoeman, F (ed), *Philosophical Dimensions of Privacy: An Anthology* (Cambridge: Cambridge UP, 1984), p 223 (slightly modified).

19 Fried, *op cit*, p 482.

20 Fried, *ibid*, p 483.

21 Fried, *ibid*, p 493.

22 Allen, A, *Uneasy Access* (Totowa: Rowman & Littlefield, 1988), p 3 (emphasis mine); cf Newell, B *et al*, "Privacy in the Family", in Roessler, B, & Mokrosinska, D (eds) *Social Dimensions of Privacy: Interdisciplinary Perspectives* (Cambridge: Cambridge UP, 2015).

23 Solove, *op cit* (2002), p 1110.

24 Marmor, A, "What Is the Right to Privacy?" *Philosophy and Public Affairs* 43[1] (2015), *passim*.

25 *ibid*, p 6 (emphasis mine).

26 Fried, *op cit*, p 484.

27 *ibid*, p 490.

28 Wright Clayton, E *et al*, "The Law of Genetic Privacy: Applications, Implications, and Limitations", *Journal of Law and the Biosciences* 6[1] (2019), p 2.

29 iibid, p 36.

30 Marmor, *op cit*, p 14.

31 cf Allen, *op cit*, ch. 5.

32 Rubold, B, & Wilson, J, "Privacy Rights and Public Information", *The Journal of Political Philosophy* 27[1] (2019), p 10; cf Frowe, H, & Parry, J, "Wrongful Observation", *Philosophy and Public Affairs* 47[1] (2019), p 128.

33 Marmor, *op cit*, p 24.

34 Marmor, *op cit*, p 21.

35 Marmor, *op cit*, p 18.

36 Even if we happen to think that people planning a walk ought to consider the possibility that they will stumble across nude bathers who think they are unobserved, and that it would be negligent not to do so, it doesn't follow that they ought not to take the risk and go for the walk anyway. Similarly, if we allow (for the sake of the argument) that Gerry was in some way negligent in not considering his brother's privacy, it doesn't follow that he ought not to have had the test: only that he ought to have thought more about his brother's privacy before doing so.

37 By analogy, driving too fast may be wrong, but there is nobody whose right is violated.

38 Though legal stipulations are not central to my argument here, it is perhaps relevant to note that Article 8 of the EU's Charter of Fundamental Rights states both that (1) "[e]veryone has the right to the protection of personal data concerning him or her", and that (2) "[e]veryone has the right of access to data which has been collected concerning him or her". Though privacy is not named in the article, these stipulations, it is fair to say, follow the contours of reasonably straightforward intuitions about privacy.

39 Marmor, *op cit*, p 5.

40 Marmor, *op cit*, p 17; emphasis mine.

41 Brassington, I, *Bioscience and the Good Life* (London: Bloomsbury, 2013), *passim*.

5 Other Ways to Think about Privacy Rights

i. Pulling and Pushing

Something that unites the accounts of privacy considered so far is that they all refer most obviously to situations in which one person would be engaged in some kind of activity to obtain information about another, the referent – to "pull" it into the interpersonal domain. Of course, if the referent is concerned to protect their privacy, they will be pulling back, trying to keep that information *out* of the interpersonal domain. Thus the paparazzo is pulling information about the starlet out into a domain other than that which it would occupy by default, and for her to try to stop the photographs being publicised would be for her to try to pull the information or control over it back to herself. My having a genetic test pulls information about my parents and siblings to me that might never otherwise have been brought to me, while their attempts to stop me are analogous to their pulling back; likewise with Gerry and Terry. For this reason, I shall classify the accounts considered so far as *pull accounts*.

An approach to understanding privacy suggested by Graeme Laurie might be characterised as being a "push" account. It is an account that begins with something like the right to be let alone, but that takes it in a different direction. We can begin here with the observation that "privacy" can relate to spatial separateness, and that an account of privacy that does not include this is incomplete:

> Frequently, privacy is conceived of as being concerned with (control of) personal information. This is informational privacy, and it is undeniably an important feature of our private sphere, but it is inadequate to explain the totality of the private sphere. To be in a state of privacy – a genuine state of separateness from others – is also to enjoy *spatial privacy*, i.e., psychological separateness from others. This can occur through disconnectedness from others (having a "private moment") *or through non-connectedness with others, such as being in a state of ignorance about one's own health.*[1]

DOI: 10.4324/9781003312512-8

If this is correct, my privacy rights will involve not only my being able to keep information about myself from others – my being able to pull it back – but also my not having it foisted upon me. I can push it away. A privacy right therefore implies a right to remain in ignorance: giving someone information about themselves that they do not want would be a violation of their separation from others, and hence of their privacy. There is in the Laurevian account a callback to Warren and Brandeis's concerns about the importance of having some "retreat from the world". If the right to privacy is the right to be let alone, then any instance in which we are not let alone would be at least a potential breach of privacy. And the Laurevian account of privacy as a push could fit reasonably comfortably with Access-to-Self accounts, provided we were willing to construe being given information the existence of which was unknown, or the content of which is undesired, as having had one's self accessed by others: they would have crossed the moat that privacy rights imply one may dig around oneself.

In this context, making an appeal to push-privacy may on the face of it appear to give us a way to handle certain otherwise-puzzling claims in the literature about privacy rights and duties. For example, Anita Allen has suggested that a person who sends unwanted and sexually-suggestive images to others over social media "violate[s] a moral duty to himself to protect his own privacy as a matter of self-care and self-respect".[2] Allen seems here to be too quick to treat one's *reasons* to care about things like self-respect as *duties*. Inasmuch as that I have defined the private as being that which is not in the interpersonal domain, there could be a way to say that a person violates the requirements of a proper concern for privacy by sharing such images; and there will be all kinds of way in which we could say that there was a duty not to send them. But whether the duty was owed (even *inter alios*) to the sender, which would imply that the sender had a right against himself that they not be sent, is not nearly so straightforward a matter. All the same, a push account of privacy might allow us to say that there has been a violation of a right of privacy – except that the right is not the sender's, but the recipient's. Information that would otherwise have remained in the domain of the private would have been forced into the interpersonal, and unwontedly: her push-privacy would thereby have been violated.

Admittedly, this is something of a challenge to how we would normally think of violations of privacy, and in some ways it might appear not to fit easily with the private-confidential-secret-taboo schema that I outlined in chapter 2. On the face of it, being told something that you have made it clear you do not want to hear may seem to belong more neatly under the heading of harassment, rather than a breach of privacy – and even then, it would only be harassment if the attempts to give information were made in bad faith and aggressively: there is quite a high bar to be crossed for something to be harassment, and trying to persuade someone that there exists some information that we really think they should know for their own sake would be likely to fall quite a long way short of it. Equally, when it comes to Allen's example, though an appeal to push-privacy does capture the general tenor of the wrong better than Allen's own account, it still seems to me that we would naturally be more inclined to treat the sender's behaviour as an instance of harassment rather than as a violation of privacy. If this is correct, then it seems to count against the push account: it is much more parsimonious not to try to find a way to fit privacy around something for which there is already a perfectly good moral description. Harassment may violate a person's privacy rights, but it does so incidentally, and we get a full-enough moral picture without having to go beyond noting an instance of harassment.

There is a tension between the push account of privacy and the CoPI account, too: an agent may exert some control over personal information when he is unaware of its content – in effect, making it taboo for himself; but it is much less clear that he would be able to exercise control over personal information when he had resisted knowing of its very existence. There would also be a puzzle about what precisely would be protected by a supposed privacy right understood this way: if someone is approaching me with information about myself that I do not want, then they already know something about me. The information somehow must have got into the interpersonal domain – perhaps my geneticist had been too talkative – and so at least as far as my privacy is concerned, it would be natural to say that the damage had been done.

ii. Push Normativity

Since defining privacy and separating it from related concepts is insufficient to ground a claim about a *right* to privacy, whether an acknowledged viola-tion of privacy implies a violation of rights to privacy and is thereby wrongful is a further question. ("Harassment" behaves slightly differently: wrongfulness is built into that word, because were an action not the kind of thing that we thought wrongful, we would not be inclined to call it harassment.) Settling the normative question may require saying whether the violation was opti-mific, but it may require more than that; and it may be important to consider the circumstances, the nature of the information, the character of the person telling the information, the manner in which it is told, and so on. It would also be necessary to consider the difference between contacting someone to tip them off that there is information that it may be worth their while tracking down, and giving them that information directly. There may be times when we would consider it better not to tell someone something that may nevertheless be very germane to their life and how they live it, or even to hide from them the fact that there is something that could be known. The truth about Cal and Aron Trask's mother is an open secret around Salinas in *East of Eden*, but it is not (at least for the bulk of the novel) quite open to the boys themselves – and this may have been for the best.[3] The knowledge of what happened to Cathy, and of what is in their lineage, does them little good; and it may be that, at least as far as that detail went, it would have been better had they been let alone. That said, nobody in Salinas keeps the information from the boys out of respect for their privacy rights. Their not being told about Cathy was more a case of keeping something secret from them, and this lesson may apply more widely. Equally, it may be difficult to assert rights in respect of push-privacy, since it will often only be possible to decide whether one wants to know something once one knows it, or at least that it is there to know.

More generally, being told something, even something that we have indicated we would prefer not to be told, by someone who tells us out of a genuine concern for our welfare does seem sometimes not to be culpable, or at least to be somewhat forgivable. Of course, there is no reason to suppose that a willingness to forgive a violation will justify that violation *post hoc*: that someone does not mind their privacy having been violated will not show that it was not violated, and there is a sense in which forgiveness implies a wrong – where there is no wrong, there is nothing to forgive. The narrator of *Green Eggs and Ham* has his push-privacy invaded by Sam-I-Am (whose actions are tantamount to harassment), and though he is by the end of the story glad to have learned something about himself and is able to reframe his behaviour in respect of the titular foodstuff, we could still criticise Sam-I-Am at least for his approach.[4] All the same, there is something attractive to the idea that a person cannot be wronged by being told something true about himself, especially if it is reasonable to think that it would be of great import to him, and if he is told without harassment. There may be a violation of push-privacy, but it does not follow that violating it is a wrong.

The lesson for genetic information ought to be clear: Gerry's telling Terry about his genome when Terry has said that he would prefer not to be told may be a violation of Terry's push-privacy, and potentially of a right. There is any number of papers in the literature arguing the pros and cons of revealing genetic information to relatives, given normal concerns about patient confidentiality. However, the overwhelming assumption that motivates these papers is that relatives would welcome warnings; the question is invariably one of whether the presumed benefit would be worth the violation of the putative rights of the one tested. This is perfectly understandable; but if Laurie's account has merit, then it looks as though there is something missing. Few consider this problem from the point of view of the privacy of the people told.

As we saw in chapter 3, Harris and Keywood have suggested that there cannot be a right to ignorance that is based in autonomy, because ignorance vitiates autonomy. If they are right, then that would seem to imply that I cannot claim that being given information is a violation of my privacy rights: "[while] the scope of privacy is indeed broad, it is difficult to argue that ignorance, a state of non-knowledge, is instrumental in the furtherance of any of the values that underpin the right to privacy".[5] Although Harris and Keywood do not think that this gives the green light to forcing information on people – information is a requirement of autonomy rather than a duty – this cannot be because there is a right to any-thing like push-privacy. Put another way: to the extent that rights to privacy are rights to remain in ignorance, privacy rights may be inimical to very thing that is supposed to mark us out as agents, and therefore rights-holders, at all.

At the other end of the scale, Husted has suggested that a properly rich account of autonomy would force us to admit that there *is* a right to privacy understood as a push – understood, that is, as a very deep right not to know genetic information about oneself. In essence, his claim is that autonomy is a matter not just of being able to make informed decisions about this or that matter, but of being able to create oneself wholesale: to decide, and to be master of, the kind of life that one lives. And for this reason

> the matter of the unsolicited disclosure of genetic findings to unsuspecting relatives begins to present itself as quite problematic. Taking the decision of whether to know or not to know out of the person's hands is a case of doing the wrong thing, being a clear case of the usurpation of decision making.[6]

Whereas Laurie's claim is that privacy entails a right to turn down the option of knowing about our genomes, such as (for example) if we tell someone that they might consider getting a genetic test because of something we have learned about a blood relative, Husted's suggestion is that true respect for autonomy would require being able to reject knowing even that there is something to know: merely approaching someone to recommend that they get a test would represent a violation of the autonomy that privacy is sup-posed to protect. Even if the person we warn chooses to ignore the warning, he contends, in having warned them at all, we will have made an ineradicable difference to their lives, and so interfered with their autonomy: "nothing will ever be the same again".[7]

iii. Assessing Push-Privacy

What should we make of push-privacy in the genetic context? Even putting aside questions of rights – and the supposed wrongness and forgivability of telling someone information they do not want – the possibility that Terry would lose privacy *qua* control over personal information should he be told something irrespectively of, or in defiance of, his wishes is a rather perplexing one. The kinds of concerns that arise from an account like Laurie's fly in the face of at least some of the received medico-ethical and medicolegal wisdom on autonomy and paternalism, which holds that autonomy requires infor-mation and that therefore respect for autonomy presupposes that agents have at least some information. As we saw in chapter 1, the received wisdom surrounding information is a part of what I have called the "standard model", under which things like privacy and confidentiality are important insofar as that they reflect a principle of autonomy.

But the content of the received wisdom is not in itself a reason to accept or to reject the received wisdom.

There is a (rightful) suspicion of withholding information from another, since that could well indicate a desire to influence that other's behaviour; and the idea that one cannot truly exercise control over one's life if one does not have at least a reasonable grasp of pertinent information is also important. Even if we disagree about what information is required for the sake of autonomous action, the proposition that *some* is appears robust: without it, an agent would be anchorless. As Rosamond Rhodes has suggested,

> when I choose to remain ignorant of relevant information, I am choosing to leave whatever happens to chance. I am following a path without autonomy. Now, if autonomy is the ground for my right to determine my own course, it cannot also be the ground for not determining my own course. If autonomy justifies my right to knowledge, it cannot also justify my refusing to be informed.[8]

For sure, if a person refuses information, the only person withholding it is the person himself, and that does make a difference: one cannot wrong oneself. But – to reprise the metaphor from a moment ago – it is also plausible to think that when it comes to the relationship between privacy and autonomy, there is an important difference between digging a moat to keep out the barbarians, and digging a moat to keep out the postman.

This perplexity invites questions about whether a right to genetic privacy, understood as a push, is all that sustainable an idea. But even if we think it is, the normative aspects raise questions of their own. Granted for the sake of the argument that telling someone something that they do not want to hear is in some way a violation of their privacy, is it wrongful? This is not obvious.

For one thing, a view like Husted's would require a radical shift in our thinking about privacy. This is not in itself a reason to resist the view; but the burden of proof is on its proponents, and there are reasons to think it quite weighty. Note, for example, the appeal to "unsolicited" genetic findings in respect of autonomy. How, though, would a person be expected to solicit findings without some sense that there were findings to solicit in the first place, and might that in itself violate the privacy of the relative who has had a genetic test? And what would the rights of the relative who had the test be? Could she refuse to disclose her results, or even that she had had a test, citing her own privacy? That, after all, would also impact the protagonist's "deep" autonomy, because any situation in which two agents can be said to be in any kind of relationship to each other will be one in which one's decisions will have *some* impact on the other. This is not a problem, or grounds to raise objections: it's a bare fact about human interaction. Relatedly, it is not at all clear that a person really is any more autonomous without unsolicited tips-off than they would be with. Granted, a tip-off about genetic risk probably will change the recipient's self-definition and be a kind of paternalism – but if that is a problem, then we have to accept that persons do nevertheless exist in the world alongside other persons, and that all benevolent interactions will be subject to the same criticism, and that if that is a moral problem we seem to be heading for a world in which the supposed vice of paternalism could be avoided only by recasting virtuous and workaday human activity as suspiciously vicious. This I take to be absurd. In fact, it would probably destroy the very autonomy we seek to preserve anyway, since agents pro-tected from the kinds of external influence that worry Husted would not obviously be able to interact meaningfully with the world at all. My decision to approach my twin with genetic information will make a difference to his autonomy – for sure, nothing will ever be the same again; but my not approaching him might be said to have the same effect, because nothing will ever be different.

Laurie himself builds a similar rebuttal of Husted's position, pointing out that it glosses unhelpfully over the difference between "prior-expressed choices not to know and no choices at all", and that choosing not to warn a person about their possible genetic profile is itself a kind of choice, and so, presumably, liable to the same kind of concerns about paternalism as telling them: *tu quoque*.[9] This point aside, a Laurevian account will not be derailed by the kind of problems raised by Husted: since this account makes no claim about the centrality of autonomy, adherents are able to accept that privacy and autonomy may both be goods, but that we can think of them apart from each other. Laurie's claim is not that we value privacy or re-cognise a right to privacy as a means of protecting autonomy – or, at least, not solely so. Such a picture fails to recognise that one of the things we want from privacy is simply separateness from others.[10] This may well be true – at least some of the time.

However, Laurie's account does still shift the emphasis of questions about privacy somewhat, so that they are no longer simply about the referent of a given piece of information: they also concern those around him. Again, this is not in itself a reason to reject push-privacy as a con-ceptual or normative position. Still, genetic privacy on this account would only stretch as far as having a right positively to reject the possibility of accessing information – it would not stretch to a right not to be told that there is information to be accessed, and it certainly would not tell us anything about rights to be told or to know – and thereby about rights to privacy in the sense that I have been considering it so far. In other words, the push account is one way of talking about informational privilege, inasmuch as that that gives us the ability to take or leave information about us as we please; but it does not really touch on the other aspect of informational privilege, which concerns our entitlement to grant or deny to others access to information of which we are the referent.

This means that a case such as ABC is left untouched by push accounts of privacy – ABC's claim was that she should have been informed about XX's diagnosis, not that she should not: it is XX's privacy that is in question rather than hers – and neither are the reasons we might have to share information with another person, or to complain that others did not share information with us.

What a push account offers us is a deeper understanding of the standard model of bioethics. This is fine – but it does not really get to grips with the importance of the distinction between confined and unconfined information; rather, it assumes that genetic testing represents just one more way in which information about a person may come to light. Since my contention is that the standard model of bioethics is not all that good at dealing with the peculiarities of unconfined information, the particular problems that unconfinement presents remain untouched.

iv. Eliminativism and Reductionism

It would be impossible to guarantee that the brief survey of ways to make sense of genetic privacy rights offered over the last chapter and a half is comprehensive. There is always going to be a chance that an account of privacy rights that can be applied convincingly to the case of genetic information is just around the corner. All the same, insofar as that the main accounts of what a privacy right would be turn out not to have much grip in respect of *genetic* information, it does look increasingly as though the concept of a right to genetic privacy may be hard to keep hold of. Even attempting to shift our focus from a pull account to a push will not really tell us all that much about who may access what and under what circumstances (although to be fair to push accounts, neither do they pretend to be able to). And on that basis, it may look as though we should strike rights to genetic privacy from our conceptual framework.

This kind of thought may come across as an invitation to eliminativism, and the expunging of phrases such as "genetic privacy rights" from the language. I have no desire to take such a radical position. Not every phrase that has a useful role to play in a natural language has a precise extension; and, for reasons that I shall set out in the final two chapters, I think that it is possible (and perhaps even desirable) to keep the language of privacy rights in respect of genetic information, albeit with some qualifications. Short of eliminativism, though, one may be inclined to a form of reductionism about genetic privacy rights: the idea would be that a term like "genetic privacy rights" is actually a metonym for rights in respect of other considerations, and that we can therefore (if we are so inclined) reduce the putative right to these other *echt* rights. In effect, a "right to genetic privacy" would be a bundle of other rights, in rather the same way that a first-order right to property is fully explicable as a bundle of second-order rights to use, to destroy, to bequeath, to alienate, and to exclude others from the use of some item.[11] If this approach is correct, it may mean we need not worry too much about a difficulty in applying privacy rights to genetic information; we ought instead to look to whatever the relevant considerations are for which the phrase "genetic privacy rights" stands, and see how they apply. Perhaps none of these higher-order rights is able to give us what we want in respect of genetic privacy; but we would at any rate be clearer on the matter than we had been, and with luck we would have dissolved the paradoxes of informational privilege along the way.

A version of this kind of reductionism is offered by Judith Jarvis Thomson in her essay "The Right to Privacy", which I shall take to be paradigmatic of the reductionist approach. Her contention is that talk about privacy rights does something that can be reduced to other kinds of right; correspondingly, what we call "privacy rights" are manifestations of, and are derivative of, higher-order rights. Broadly speaking, these higher-order rights are rights "that certain steps shall not be taken to find out facts, and [rights] that certain uses shall not be made of facts".[12] Obviously, if Thomson is successful in her attempt to reduce privacy rights across the board, *genetic* privacy rights will be subject to the same kind of reduction; but even if privacy rights *sensu lato* cannot be reduced, we might still be able to perform the reductionist trick in respect of genetic privacy rights.

The nub of Thomson's argument is that privacy rights are in one way comparable to rights that one has over one's body; to have a privacy right is an extension of a right that we have not to be looked at, or listened to, or touched. Such rights are gathered under the umbrella term "right over the person".[13] Privacy rights are in another way comparable to property rights: "the right to not be looked at and the right to not be listened to are analogous to rights we have over our property",[14] inasmuch as that when we claim that a person who looks at a picture we own violates a right we have – a right that we would normally call a privacy right – that it not be looked at.[15] Ultimately,

> [i]t begins to suggest itself, then, as a simplifying hypothesis, that the right to privacy is itself a cluster of rights, and that it is not a distinct cluster of rights but itself intersects with the cluster of rights which the right over the person consists in and also with the cluster of rights which owning property consists in.[16]

Correspondingly, my right that someone not look at my medical records might be couched as a claim about a privacy right, but that phrasing would turn out to be simply a way of talking about other rights; and I have a right to privacy inasmuch as that, and for whatever reason that, I have a right for those records not to be examined, or perhaps even seen.[17] A violation of privacy is wrong for the same reasons that using a x-ray goggles to look into someone's safe is wrong; and that is because our bodies, like our possessions, are *ours*.

Still, privacy rights are reducible to rights over one's person or over one's property only if there is *no* privacy right that is not at the same time a right over one's person or over one's property. If there is any such "independent" privacy right – if there is just one instance in which we would be inclined to talk about a privacy right in a way that is not reducible to some other kind of right, irrespective of whatever huge number of instances it is in which such reduction is possible – all we will have is a situation in which there are certain family resemblances between privacy rights and other kinds of right, and in which they sometimes overlap. So, for example, if we spy on a person in order to learn what he does in his kitchen at midnight, we violate a right not to be looked at, "which is both one of the rights which the right to privacy consists in and one of the rights which the right over the person consists in".[18] But this would not show that privacy rights are reducible: all it shows is that there are certain violations that could easily be described as belonging to one or both of two sets.

But Thomson is inclined to think that there is in fact no instance of a putative privacy right that is not reducible to some other kind of right. Thus she moots the idea that "doing something to a man to get personal information from him is violating his right to privacy only if doing that to him is violating some right of his not identical with or included in the right to privacy".[19] For Thomson, then, if we are inclined to say that (say) torturing or eavesdropping on a person to learn information about him violates his privacy, it does so only insofar as that we are torturing or eavesdropping on him. Merely learning something about him in a way that does not violate some other right would not, she holds, count as violating a right to privacy. And so she summarises her position thus:

> We have a right to not be tortured. Why? Because we have a right to not be hurt or harmed. I have a right that my pornographic picture shall not be torn. Why? Because it's mine, because I own it. I have a right to do a somersault now. Why? Because I have a right to liberty. I have a right to try to preserve my life. Why? Because I have a right to life. In these cases we explain the having of one right by appeal to the having of another which includes it. *But I don't have a right to not be looked at because I have a right to privacy*; I don't have a right that no one shall torture me in order to get personal information about me because I have a right to privacy; *one is inclined, rather, to say that it is because I have these rights that I have a right to privacy.*[20]

Thomson's claim is that, at least *qua* right, there is not much going on with privacy at all: the scope and content of a putative right to privacy are unclear to her, and she admits that there seems to her to be "much slithering in the literature" on the topic.[21] Her position is superficially similar to a control account, whether that be control of access to the self or of access to personal information. The difference is that, under her account, we can do away with appeals to privacy and the language of privacy if we are so inclined, because there is nothing in the concept of a right to privacy that cannot be understood in terms of rights of ownership, rights over ourselves, rights not to be caused distress, rights not to be caused annoyance, and so on. So, sure: talk about rights to privacy, or privacy rights. But don't go thinking that we are thereby talking about something *sui generis*, because we aren't. Talk about privacy rights is possible because it is a product of talk about higher-order rights.

Yet this position as it stands leaves out something important about putative privacy rights. Thomson holds that a right to privacy can be understood in terms of "a right that certain uses shall not be made of facts".[22] But (I would contend) a violation of privacy does not require that any use be made of the information: it is enough that it be brought into the interpersonal realm. She is also slightly vulnerable to the objection that she is making life too easy for herself in that, by not offering a definitive list of higher-order rights that the right to privacy may represent, it becomes very difficult for a notional opponent to present a counter-example: Thomson's claim would resist falsification because new higher-order rights could be added to the list *ad hoc* and indefinitely. Equally, for any number of candidate explanations of the putative right to privacy that one might offer, there is always potentially another higher-order right, possibly with more explanatory power, that has not been considered. This does not undermine the essence of the reductionist claim; but it does mean that we may have to accept that what we're reducing putative privacy rights to could be indeterminate. And the danger with this is that the reductionist may be liable to think that an inability to show what a putative right to privacy reduces to is unimportant when trying to convince others of the truth of reductionism. It may not be.

Still, the important point is that an account such as Thomson's might help us clarify some of the ways in which the language of privacy is and ought to be used. Reductionism does not mean that genetic privacy is a boojum; but it does mean that we have to think carefully about what, exactly, is going on with the problems that we associate with it.

v. Reductionism and Genetic Information

So what would we be invited to think about genetic privacy if a reductionist account is correct? We do not have to be able to give a definitive account of which rights are engaged in order to make progress; and there is a number of higher-order rights of which a right to genetic privacy may be an avatar. The most likely candidates are rights not to be known, and rights not to be harmed. Each of these is, in its way, a kind of right over access to the self, or to what I called in the last chapter the extended self, and so would appear to slot into a model like the AtS account quite nicely, and perhaps to bolster it. I shall deal with a right not to be harmed first.

One of the most intuitively attractive accounts of what is going on with a first-order privacy right would surely run along the lines that privacy matters (including in respect of genetic information) because it is protective in at least a couple of ways. First, that certain things are known may be directly harmful. "Harm" in this telling should be taken quite widely, so that it encompasses not only being made materially worse off, but also lost opportunities, stigmatisation, and so on. Second, it may be indirectly harmful, in that information that is accessible might leave us vulnerable to harms such as blackmail. As such, a right to genetic privacy would imply protection against quite a wide range of things. And yet if this is the kind of line that we want to take, it is not certain that it would quite give us what we would generally want from a privacy right; and if that is right, then privacy rights would not be reducible to rights against being harmed alone.

The reason for this caution is that, when people talk about privacy, they *may* have in mind its importance for the sake of avoiding harm – but they may not. For example, the starlet on whose window the paparazzo has his camera trained is not harmed by that except insofar as that he does have his camera trained on the window. An account that tries to reduce the violation of her right to privacy to a right not to be harmed would struggle to deal with this – for in what would the harm consist *except* that she had had her privacy violated? Were the images captured to generate some further harm, there may be a different story to tell: but on the twin assumptions that his spying on her is opportunistic and that he sees nothing that is in any way remarkable, stigmatised, or stigmatising (and is therefore unlikely to be a subject ripe for blackmail), then the story will not obviously go much further. And so if the right to privacy is reducible to, or explicable in terms of, a right not to be harmed, then many of the things that one might expect to be covered by privacy rights would turn out not to be.

Admittedly, my wide definition of harm leaves some scope for a comeback along the lines that maybe the harm suffered by the starlet is bare embarrassment. We can allow that embarrassment is a kind of harm, broadly speaking, since it is the kind of state that a person might rationally wish to avoid irrespective of whether there is any further harm. Neither does something have to be shameful for its discovery to be a source of embarrassment. Suppose the starlet has a habit of putting on music dancing really rather badly when she thinks that nobody is looking. There is nothing shameful about this; but she might be embarrassed by it all the same. Equally, you may be embarrassed if I see (or if you think I have seen) your bank statement, irrespective of what it says. Presumably, the same may apply in respect of the information stored in our genomes. And so if a right to privacy is a right not to be harmed, and embarrassment is a kind of harm, and we may be embarrassed by certain information, and some of that information may be genetic in nature, then it looks as though we could say that there are grounds for a claim about a right to genetic privacy.

Nevertheless, it is not clear how much further we can go with this line of reasoning. The most obvious confounding consideration is that there may be times when a person has a defensible interest in accessing information the referent of which is another person, even if the referent could or would be harmed in some way thereby. Some actions may be justifiable all things considered, notwithstanding that they do generate some harms; and there is therefore no sustainable right that they not be done. For example, taxation leaves us worse off than we might conceivably have been, and is something that we might rationally prefer to avoid, and so counts as a harm on the wide interpretation I am allowing here – yet we can admit this at the same time as admitting that it is justified all things considered, and that harm will not give us a right not to be (fairly) taxed. As such, it may be that agents have reasons to prefer that other agents avoid some harmful things; but it does not follow that it would be wronged if they faced those harms all the same. No right seems to have been jeopardised. We may have rights that protect us from harmful things, but this does not mean that we have rights that protect us from *all* harmful things. And so if a right to privacy is to be understood in this way, it probably reduces to a right not to be harmed *gratuitously* or *needlessly*. But harming people, or making them susceptible to harm, gratuitously or needlessly is plainly something that we ought not to do anyway, and so it is not clear what appeals to *ab initio* privacy rights add to the mix, except to get in the way of our gaining access to information to which we may have some plausible claim.

Neither is it obvious why genetic information would be exempt from this principle. Sooner or later, we will come up against the idea that there could be times when one person (such as Gerry) has a morally defensible reason to access information about another or his genome even though there is some sense in which access may harm that second person (such as Terry) insofar as that it sets back a particular interest of his. At such a time, though there might be a case for Gerry not being allowed access to that information, it would be a case that Terry would have to make rather than one that he could take as a given. The agent who seeks access may have the more powerful claim. In fact, this point has particular piquancy when it comes to genetic information: even if we want to reject genetic exceptionalism as a normative principle, we have to accept that unconfined information behaves differently from confined. There may be times – as in the case of close relatives having access to genetic information – when the supposed harm (perhaps manifesting as embarrassment) arising from having information about one's genome known to others must be balanced against a presumably equally worrisome harm that accrues to them from *not* having access to it. Their inability simply to know themselves may count as a kind of harm, as might the loss of opportunity to act in respect of unrevealed genetic timebombs. Importantly, because genetic information is unconfined, one of the parties will face some harm one way or another. Neither is this point restricted to identical twins like Gerry and Terry: it applies to any persons – Benny, Jenny, Kenny, Lenny, and Penny – whose genomes overlap significantly. Either way, even if this is a harm arising from information entering the interpersonal domain, we cannot infer from that that there is any right engaged, because not all harms generate protective rights. There is an indefinitely large number of things that may be harmful without violating any credible right.

What Benny would have to show in order to keep Penny from accessing putatively private information is that any harm incurred is the sort of thing that does generate a right to privacy. Any agent's blood relations may worry that that agent's having a genetic test will tell him something about them, or those (such as children) whose interests they have a duty to protect. And yet an incidental finding about someone else's genome may be embarrassing for that other, and it may be in some other sense harmful; however, that is not going to tell us anything about anyone's rights to require that the test not be taken. I would contend that establishing a right is likely to be difficult – difficult enough in respect of conventional medical information, but especially so in the case of genetic information. (Naturally, this will tell us nothing about non-relatives' attempts to access information. I shall consider these in the next chapter.)

Furthermore, there are reasons to think that putative rights to genetic privacy would be particularly hard to protect by appeals to embarrassment, because the very idea of embarrassment is subject to scrutiny from a number of directions. The supposed harm arising from embarrassment is unlike the harm that we might think could arise when material interests are set back: the fact of that person's being embarrassed is not all that normatively hefty, since there are times when we could plausibly say that a person who is embarrassed nevertheless *ought not* to be. No fault is implied by being the carrier of this or that gene, and there is little that one could do about it anyway. We might therefore be inclined to think that any embarrassment that a person may feel about his genome would be unwarranted and therefore not all that big a normative consideration. This is a response that does not even require sacrificing any sensitivity to the fact of a person's embarrassment. In fact, discovering that one shares a gene with another – or being discovered to share it – is at least as plausibly a basis for a sense of solidarity as embarrassment.

And so the idea that a right to privacy reduces to a right not to be harmed would seem to be vulnerable to attack on a number of fronts. Having information brought into the public realm *may* violate a right not to be harmed, say by leaving us vulnerable to exploitation, or simply by being embarrassing; but it is not always going to do that, and even if harm accrues, its moral importance will have to be weighed against the harm of others' lost opportunities. This implies that we would have to say either that there is no right to privacy engaged when there is no real prospect of harm, or that reducing a right to privacy to a right not to be harmed does not tell the full story. It is at this point that the other putative source of a right to privacy comes into play: that a right to privacy is not (just) a right not to be harmed, but is a right not to be known at all.

Suppose I take a look at your bank statement, and thereby learn that you are neither rich nor poor, but unremarkably comfortable. You would not really be harmed by this, nor opened to harm; if there is a wrong here, it lies just in the fact that I have sought out something about you and your extended self that I ought not to have sought out, and that it is this kind of wrong against which a right to privacy articulates a defence. It is likely that we care about privacy insofar as that information's having been accessed at all represents a violation of our boundaries, over which we would be inclined to claim certain rights of control. Similarly, we would seem to be able to say that the voyeur wrongs those on whom he spies without having to say that they have been caused any particular harm – and if there has been a harm, then that could quite plausibly be explained by the damage caused by knowing that they had been wronged: the knowledge that one's boundaries have been violated that may be upsetting, but the wrong of having one's boundaries violated would be primary, and would persist irrespective of whether or not one knew about or was particularly fussed by it.

At first glance, it seems that this goes for genetic information as much as it goes for any other kind of information, its having been brought into the interpersonal realm plausibly wronging the referent, irrespective of any harm done. There may be a wrong even when there is a good prospect of benefit: for example, if identifiable genetic information found its way into medical research that ended up helping the referent, then that referent may admit that they are in some way better off, but could coherently claim to have been wronged all the same.

Still, the shortcoming of an account that relies on a right not to be known as an explanation for privacy rights ought to be fairly clear when it comes to explaining intuitions about genetic privacy (particularly, though not exclusively, when we are considering people who are closely related), and that is – again – because genetic information is unconfined. A right to remain unknown would necessarily run up against the wall of other rights that we presumably would want to take seriously: rights such as a right to know oneself. Echoing the argument of chapter 3, if we were to bite the bullet and accept that the wrong of having one's genome discovered gives others a reason, even one that falls short of being a duty, to remain in ignorance about their genomes, it would turn out that everyone has the same reason – which would mean that we were not talking about privacy after all, so much as about something much more like a taboo. We would be less the owners of our genetic information than its prison guards. But if it is impossible for one person to know himself or his genome without coming to know others, it would not be obvious that there would be any wrong in knowing about another's genome (or the statistical likelihood that a non-identical relative has a particular trait) – and therefore that there would be any right not to be known. And there is any number of instances, inside or outside of the genetic realm, when one person might come to know something about another without there having been any wrong. This claim does not undermine the idea aired in chapter 2 that one may have a duty to try to forget things unwittingly learned.

Just as a supposed right not to be placed in a harmed position turned out to be likely to mean a right not to be placed *gratuitously* in such a position, it strikes me that the putative right not to be known, understood in its broad sense, would best be thought of as generating a moral defence against being *pried upon* rather than a right to be known (or seen, or sensed in some other way) at all. It is important in this respect to note that not all instances in which one comes to know information about another, even deliberately, is properly called an instance of prying: to pry implies an element of prurience.[23] One can be seen, or come to be known, without being pried upon; and one can see or come to know without prurience. We can say that if Gerry has a genetic test in order to learn something about his brother, then there may be a violation of Terry's privacy. But for Gerry to have learning about his brother as the rationale for his test would be odd, to say the least, and we would not need to make any appeal to Terry's rights to launch an entirely cogent moral criticism of Gerry's actions. In a more plausible arrangement of affairs, Gerry's having a genetic test will mean that Terry's genome may become "visible" to Gerry (and this may even be the sort of thing that Terry regards as harmful). Still, if Gerry finds out about his brother's genome in the course of finding out about his own, then this is the equivalent of *seeing* Terry, not of *looking at* him. Gerry has a reason (and quite possibly a duty) not to pry on his brother, in roughly the same way that he as a reason (and quite possibly a duty) not to harm him arbitrarily or gratuitously; but if that is all that there is to a right to privacy, there is not all that much. Importantly, the moral focus will be on Gerry's motivations, rather than on Terry's supposed rights.

Equally, a right not to be pried upon clearly does not imply a right to deny others access to information of which they are at the same time the referent; in fact, as I shall argue in the next chapter, neither does it imply a blanket right to deny others access to information even when they are *not* the referent: we have to think of the interests in play more widely. And so, in the ABC case, had ABC herself suspected that her father had Huntington's and taken a genetic test to find that out, and had this been for prurient reasons, I would be inclined to say that she would have wronged XX by invading his privacy. But putting to one side the ineffectiveness of the strategy (testing oneself will tell us about a particular parent only sometimes), prurience would likely not be the motive. Whether this tells us that ABC herself had a right *to be told* is a slightly different matter, to which I shall return in chapter 8. (One important but for the moment slightly tangential question is worth raising here, and it is a version of the Euthyphro dilemma: is prying wrong because it violates a right that someone has, or do they have that right because prying is wrong? I am inclined to think that it is the latter option that we should choose, and shall say more about why in chapter 7.)

vi. Reducing Reductionism

There may be any number of higher-order rights to which a putative right to genetic privacy would be reducible. A right not to be harmed, and a right not to be known strike me as being the most obvious candidates, but there may be others. And it may be that a right to genetic privacy engages more than one higher-order right. Nevertheless, the onus would be on the defender of genetic privacy to show two things: first, that there is something to which a right to privacy reduces; and second, that that something generates a moral reason sufficiently compelling to be able to block others' access. Whether those demands can be met is uncertain. A referent's concern that he may be harmed or wronged by information being accessed by another would have to be considered in light of the harm or wrong that that other would incur by not accessing it. Adding other higher-order rights to which a privacy right may be reduced does not alter this picture; it simply means that the network of claims about higher-order rights would be that much more complicated. And if others can acknowledge that their accessing information may cause harm or simply lead to being known, this does not necessarily settle the matter, because we might still think that they have a defensible moral reason to access the information in question. This being so, a "right to genetic privacy" would turn out to reduce to very little, if anything.[24] In effect, we would be saying that the right to (genetic) privacy obtains when accessing information would be prurient or otherwise improper, or when there is no good reason for it to be accessed. But that is trivially true, and – as I said a moment ago – actually shifts the moral focus from the supposed rights-holder to the putative accessors and their motivations. In effect, for Alice to say that she has a right to privacy means that Bob has a moral reason not to access certain information because of something that lies with her; the shift means that Bob's moral reasons would have to do with something about him. I think that we should embrace this shift, and I shall develop the line of thought in chapters 7 and 8; but we should be clear about what is going on.

The endpoint of all this is that reductionism about privacy rights is not a position we should embrace too eagerly if we want to keep hold of the idea that the term "privacy right" names something morally substantial. This point stands even if the supposed right to privacy reduces to something other than a right against harm, or a right against being known – even then, whatever the right it is to which the right to privacy reduces would have to be weighed against the merits of the claims of the person seeking to access the information, or against the rights of the person who ends up "seeing" it, to do whatever it is that leads to their seeing it. Whichever way we parse things, reductionism does not get quite to the nerve of what is going on when people talk about genetic privacy, and it does not make the problems thrown up by privacy claims go away. What it *does* do is help us get a firm hold on the nature of those problems. This is no small thing.

Reductionism about privacy rights may lead us to think that we should abandon the language of privacy rights, in favour of more accurate talk about rights not to be harmed, not to be known, or whatever it may be. I think that this would be too hasty. To see why, consider the idea that our vocabulary dealing with things like colour is reducible to talk about the electromagnetic spectrum: talk about red light and green light or about microwaves or x-rays is to talk about electromagnetic waves of particular frequencies. We would not want to say that the vocabularies are mutually substitutable: we can still say that the term "red light" means a particular wavelength of electromagnetic radiation in a way that "electromagnetic radiation" does not mean "red light". By the same sort of reasoning, even if what we call "a right to privacy" turns out to be, in a sense, an avatar of other, higher-order rights, it would not follow that the language of those higher-order rights would be applicable in all situations in which the lower-order language would be applicable. In fact, it seems more likely that trying to eliminate the language of privacy would make matters *less* clear.

So the question, as it turns out, concerns *how* we deploy the language of privacy rights, not whether we deploy it at all. The position I shall adopt in the final two chapters of the book is that, if we decide in a given situation that an agent should be able to keep certain information out of the interpersonal domain or to restrict access to it because of the harm that will accrue should it be accessible, then we will *on that basis* be able to say that it is private. This is wholly in keeping with the reductionist programme: the privacy claim *per se* would not really be what was carrying the moral weight, but it would provide a way to talk neatly about the things that are. What we would not be saying is that the agent could keep access restricted *because* it is private. Again, I shall elaborate on this point a little later.

The language of privacy does things that we tend to want to be done. This is not a conclusive reason to maintain the idea, of course: if a concept makes no sense, then no amount of wishing that did would generate a reason to keep it. But doing away with the language of genetic privacy rights too hastily would leave us vulnerable to the idea that genetic information is, and could not help but to be, a free-for-all: that if an agent has no coherent privacy rights over his genome, and this is because there is no such right or – which amounts to the same thing – because there would be insuperable obstacles in spelling out what the right protects, this means that nobody has a privacy right over their genome; and that, in turn, would seem to imply that anyone could claim access to anyone else's genetic information. That that would be a position that we would presumably want to resist. We might wonder, then, where to draw the line: granted the supposition that there is *something* that imposes a limit on how much genetic information should be accessible to others, what is it?

In the next chapter, I shall probe these questions further, arguing that though there are reasons to want to keep hold of the idea of privacy, there are also reasons to allow at least some access. In particular, I shall explore the idea that, although there is a powerful intuition that nobody is under any obligation to provide genetic information to others, this intuition may not hold in all cases – and I shall use insurers' access to genetic information as the exemplar. If I am correct in this, the idea of informational privilege yielding a right to genetic privacy will be under attack on two fronts: the conceptual and the practical. The conceptual attack has been outlined in this chapter and the last: whether we are talking about the control of personal information, or access to the self or extended self, or about privacy as a pull or a push, or as representing some other right, genetic information seems a bit too slippery. But the practical attack hinges on the idea that even if we can get a tight conceptual grip on a right to genetic privacy, there may be good moral reasons to relax it. And this would mean that putative rights to genetic privacy would turn out to be simply moral reasons among other moral reasons.

Notes

1 Laurie, G, "Recognizing the Right not to Know: Conceptual, Professional, and Legal Implications", *Journal of Law, Medicine & Ethics* 42[1] (2014), p 58 (emphasis mine).

2 Allen, A, "An Ethical Duty to Protect One's Own Information Privacy", *Alabama Law Review* 64[4] (2013), p 864.

3 Steinbeck, J, *East of Eden* (London: Penguin, 2000), *passim*.

4 Seuss, Dr, *Green Eggs and Ham* (London: HarperCollins, 2016), *passim*.

5 Harris, J, & Keywood, K, "Ignorance, Information and Autonomy", *Theoretical Medicine and Bioethics* 22[5] (2001), p 430.

6 Husted, J, "Autonomy and the Right Not to Know", in Chadwick, R *et al* (eds), *The Right to Know and the Right Not to Know* (Cambridge:. Cambridge UP, 2014), p 33.

7 *ibid*, p 35.

8 Rhodes, R, "Genetic Links, Family Ties, and Social Bonds: Rights and Responsibilities in the Face of Genetic Knowledge", *The Journal of Medicine and Philosophy* 23[1] (1998), pp 10–30, p 18.

9 Laurie, G, "Privacy and the Right Not to Know: A Plea for Conceptual Clarity", in Chadwick, R *et al* (eds), *The Right to Know and the Right Not to Know* (Cambridge: Cambridge UP, 2014), p 40.

10 *ibid*, p 41.

11 cf Honoré, T, *Making Law Bind* (Oxford: Clarendon, 1987), p 165.

12 Thomson, JJ, "The Right to Privacy", *Philosophy and Public Affairs* 4[4] (1975), p 307.

13 *ibid*, p 305.

14 *ibid*, p 304.

15 *ibid*, pp 298–299.

16 *ibid*, p 306.

17 *ibid*, p 313.

18 *ibid*, pp 307–308.

19 *ibid*, p 308 (emphasis mine).

20 *ibid*, p 312 (emphasis mine).

21 *ibid*, p 285.

22 *ibid*, p 307.

23 Thomson blurs the distinction between being heard and being listened to, which leads her to suggest that being listened to need not be a violation of privacy. But this claim seems to me to be on the face of it wrong – and the scenario that she generates to set up the claim seems to me to be one in which she is talking about being *heard*, rather than *listened to*, anyway.

24 It is also notable that when Laurie is ostensibly talking about rights to privacy, the word "rights" plays a perhaps-surprisingly small role – rather, he tends to talk in terms of interests; as we shall see, this is probably the right approach.

6 Privacy and Reasons to Disclose

i. From Theories to Norms

What I have been describing so far is a number of ways in which we might attempt to provide a foundation for the idea of a right to genetic privacy, and reasons to think that they don't quite work. A violation of putative genetic privacy rights is not all that well characterised as an agent not being let alone, nor as a problem of a loss of control over access to the self or to personal information, at least where blood relatives are involved, because one person's maintaining control over genetic information must come at the expense of those relatives' having it. Reducing the idea of rights to privacy to some other kind of right may help clarify the problem and the reasons we have for thinking privacy important, but it won't make the problem go away. And trying to understand putative genetic privacy rights through the lens of push-privacy will also be of limited help.

None of this would amount to a positive, knock-down argument against rights to genetic privacy. I shall suggest in this chapter, though, that even if there does turn out to be a way to provide a conceptual foundation to intuitions about rights to genetic privacy that maintains intuitions about rights of access, there may be situations in which we ought to allow "our" information to be shared. And if that is right – if there are situations in which I ought to give you access to genetic information – then it is not clear what work a rights claim would be doing. A right that one ought not to assert is not obviously much of a right. This does not mean that there would not be any situations in which one could deny access to genetic information to others – but I shall argue that this would suggest that privacy rights are something derived on a case-by-case basis from the prevailing moral reasons, rather than things that one could bring to the table and present as fully-fledged reasons to deny access. I shall go deeper into this claim in the next two chapters.

If I am correct, it would not matter if someone came up with an explanation of the concept of privacy that was immune to the concerns raised so far, because the argument travels along a different axis. As such, "privacy rights" ought to be understood henceforward in the most general sort of way, such that a right to privacy would be a right to deny access to property or

DOI: 10.4324/9781003312512-9

information irrespective of whether that is fundamentally about rights to be let alone, or to control access to the self or to personal information, or whatever else.

ii. The Joint Account Model

It is difficult to avoid speaking as though, when it comes to genetic information, it is mine or yours to do with as I or you please, but a moment's reflection will show that matters must be more complicated than that. Information about, say, whether I had my adenoids removed as a child can be said to be "mine" because it is confined: it is about me. But genetic information is unconfined. This must make a difference.

Information's being held in common is fundamental to the "joint-account" model (JAM) of genetic information proposed by Michael Parker and Anneke Lucassen. In some ways, it echoes the information-as-property model considered in chapter 4; and though it is not quite the same as a relational-autonomy model, it suggests many of the same normative conclusions.[1] In a nutshell, the model proposes that information could, and should, be treated in a way that is analogous to the way we treat information about joint financial affairs. It is fairly common for something like a bank account to be held in common by two or more people – perhaps because they are married, or business partners. Under the JAM, blood relatives (of at least a certain proximity) can be thought of as co-holders of genetic information. As such, say Parker and Lucassen, "on the joint account model it is assumed that information should be available to all account holders unless there are good reasons to do otherwise"[2] (although this information might not include the identity of the primary referent[3]); and for an agent to stand firm on genetic information not being shared with other holders would be "analogous to me asking my bank manager not to reveal information about a joint account to my fellow account holders".[4] In passing, the JAM provides a way to respond to Loi's claim that "my genome, just like my lungs, is a part of my body [...], and I am the only person having a moral right of ownership over it"[5]: even if we think that the genome is a part of the body, it is not "just like" organs. One is host to one's genome at least as much as one is its owner; and it is far from clear that one is the *only* person with moral rights of ownership over it.

This model is rather appealing. Assuming a right to privacy in respect of genetic information obtains, it would not be something that just one person has in respect of a given piece of information. This move eliminates many of the concerns articulated over the past couple of chapters about the notionally private devolving to the secret or taboo. The moat of informational privilege will enclose not one person at a time, but several. Claims about genetic privacy *within* this moat would have to be abandoned, but they would still make perfect sense when considering who has access to what information and on what basis when one of the claimants is outside it. Just as the person who owns shares in a company cannot deny access to financial information about that company to the other shareholders, although all would have a right (and perhaps a duty) to restrict its access to the public at large, so Terry cannot use appeals to privacy to deny access to genetic information to his identical twin Gerry. Nor – in Parker and Lucassen's picture – could Lenny deny it to his sister Penny. But in both cases, there would be an indefinitely large number of other people who would violate privacy by accessing that information, and to whom Gerry, Terry, Lenny, and Penny would be perfectly within their rights to deny access to it.

Parker and Lucassen adduce a number of reasons for opting in favour of the JAM. They hold that treating genetic information as something held in a joint account reflects the way that healthcare practitioners actually do behave in the real world; and they add that treating genetic information as if it were confined to one person would mean relinquishing the opportunity for benefits (such as the opportunity to research, and potentially thereby to provide prophylaxis for, genetic illnesses) that may arise from sharing it. Moreover, for someone to discover independently that they are vulnerable to a genetic illness that could potentially have been treated earlier had medical staff who knew about their likely vulnerability informed them could do serious harm to trust in the medical profession; this could be avoided if the medics in question recognised that the genetic information in question was not the sole property of their patient, even if that patient is the primary referent. (They note too that medical staff who withhold potentially important information may also be open to legal action – a point that would obviously find an echo in the *ABC* case – although I am not particularly interested in the legal aspect here.[6]) Finally, they make an appeal to justice, noting that it is not clear why only one person should be able to benefit from genetic information that is essentially familial in nature.[7] Indeed, they go so far as to suggest that the sharing of genetic information with relevant parties should be routine.[8] This helps to soothe worries about what they claim clinical geneticists do already: it turns out to be probably the right thing; and if there are incidental benefits to be had, then so much the better.

Not all of these reasons for accepting a JAM are entirely convincing. The easiest to dismiss is the point about avoiding legal action: wanting not to be sued is a reason to act in a given way, but legal reasons will not parent conclusive moral reasons, and we cannot deduce moral principles from legal ones. Equally, tacit endorsement of something like a joint account model by clinical geneticists won't tell us whether they *ought* to endorse it. Neither does the potential loss of benefits from keeping information under wraps generate a compelling argument: a missed opportunity to derive benefits is not a harm. Indeed, there is any amount of information that is private by commonsense accounts but that we would not insist ought to be shared *pro bono publico*; genetic information would not obviously be any different. If rights are anything, they are constraints on the kinds of things that one may do to others, or to or with their possessions, even if the benefits are great; if there really is a right to genetic privacy, then the lost opportunities for benefit sharing will simply be crosses we have to bear.

The appeal to justice is somewhat heftier. There may be a concern that questions are being begged, since "justice" can be understood in several different ways, and there may be a concern that the way that the word is to be understood has been selected in order to prop up the model – and that someone with a different account of justice might want to kick out the JAM. But these concerns can be met: in pointing out that genetic information is unconfined by its nature, we can say that if deciding who has access to what genetic information and on what terms has anything to do with justice – as surely it does – we must take into account relevant facts about genetic information whatever our preferred model of justice. Correspondingly, accepting (as we should) Parker and Lucassen's point about the familial nature of genetic information will give us a way to face down complaints that sharing information violates rights of privacy or confidentiality, because it allows for a counterassertion that such complaints ignore basic facts about the information in question that make a naïve appeal to an individual's right to privacy unsustainable.

For example, Jørgen Husted's essay on autonomy and rights not to know genetic information begins with the example of a familiar dilemma in which we have to choose between giving a person genetic information that may play a role in making important life decisions, and the right to privacy of the family member from whom we derived this information.[9] But by telling us that the primary referent has a "right", and that her relatives only have interests, Husted has loaded the dice. A fair version of the question would be agnostic about whether the primary referent has a relevant right to privacy in such circumstances; and a joint-account model might well give us a reason to suppose that she doesn't.

One could pick similar faults even when the word "rights" is not used. Rhodes has denied the propriety of medical staff sharing genetic information with family members on the basis that it would violate expectations about confidentiality, which matters "because it shows respect for patient autonomy and consideration for privacy".[10] But this assumes the validity and applicability of the standard model of bioethics, and that privacy and confidentiality considerations apply to genetic information in the same way that they apply to other medical information: in other words, it assumes informational confinement. More, it risks keeping information secret from a person to whom it may be relevant. But if we are inclined to think that genetic information represents either an exception to the standard model, or a reason to modify it, then this kind of complaint is de-fanged. Bluntly, what is missing from her account is that the status of genetic information in respect of things like privacy and confidentiality is already contestable. If it is jointly held (or refers to something that is jointly held), then Rhodes's concerns are moot, because the person informed about the primary referent's genome presumably has an entitlement to it anyway based on a shared holding. And so while it may be true that "[t]he responsibilities of one family member to another do not translate into license for physicians to breach confidentiality

or to renegotiate the doctor-patient relationship with respect to confidentiality",[11] we only really need to worry about this if we are presuming that
confidentiality is in play to begin with. Arguably, it is not.

iii. Which Interests?

What is crucial in the JAM is that decisions about access to information
are to be made not simply (or even at all) by appealing to the referent and
their privacy rights, but to the interests and the justice of serving the
interest of all interested parties. This is, I think, correct, and I shall say
more about why in chapter 7. Naturally, there will be questions to ask here
about what kind of interest is in play, and who counts as an interested
party. Matthew Liao has pointed out the rather obvious point that genomes
are fully jointly-held only in a comparatively small number of cases: the
more distant the blood relationship, the less there will be in common
between parties, meaning that even fraternal twins will have significantly
different genomes. Moreover, where penetrance is low, appeals to the
desirability of prophylaxis for whatever conditions might be associated with
a gene will generate less of a pressing reason to share information. He
concludes that "the idea that genetic information is familial in nature does
not seem to provide sufficient ground for why we should move towards a
system in which by default we would share our genetic information with
our relatives".[12]

Yet this point is open to the same kind of response that I have levelled at
Rhodes: it assumes that genetic information is confined, that the standard
model is a robust way to deal with it, and that the question we should be
asking ourselves in all situations is whether a person ought to be granted
access to information that would normally be closed to them: what proximity
of relationship and what kind of interest would give us a reason to require
information-sharing. Liao's question – "Is there a duty to share genetic
information?" – is not the one that the JAM addresses, but neither is it one
that its proponents *must* address, at least directly. What the JAM does is to
allow us to suggest that *when* there is a significant overlap of "ownership" and
an interest in the information being shared, the ability of one party to limit
access to information for reasons of privacy is diluted simply because of the
kind of thing that genetic information is. Indeed, Liao's question tacitly
assumes that questions of access are predominantly concerned with situations
in which the information "belongs" to one person, who may or may not have
reasons or obligations to let others in on it. When he articulates his suspicion
about making it the default that we should share our genetic information
with relatives, the context makes it clear that it is, for him, "our" information
in the sense that a box of chocolates might be *ours*, and that decisions about
whether to share it are analogous to decisions about how generous to be with
those chocolates, rather than "ours" in the sense of being held in common. A
true joint account would not work like that.

In a related way, when Niklas Juth considers the joint account model, the question he poses is whether there is "any reason to give *special* weight to the essentially *familial* nature of *genetic* information", granted that "there are many other kinds of medical information informative of others, where we do not think it self-evident that the *default* should be sharing the information or placing little weight on confidentiality, eg, information about contagious disease". The best he can come up with to answer this question is that "we have special duties towards our blood relatives, merely due to the fact that they are our blood relatives" – a view that he thinks does not have much power.[13] But this mischaracterises the JAM. The proposal is not that we have a special reason to share information that we "own" with relatives who do not own it; it is that they already have ownership, if they only knew it. Seen this way, we don't need to worry about whether the reasons we have to share genetic information are like or unlike the reasons we have to share other kinds of information because the thing to which the information refers is already shared, and not sharing it looks rather like keeping a secret about a person from that person.

And so, *to the extent that genetic information is jointly held*, questions about rights to privacy and reasons and obligations to share are not the right questions to ask, any more than they are the right questions to ask about information flows between the joint trustees of a bank account.

But an important move has been made here. There are two ways of thinking about the legitimacy of informing people other than the primary referent of genetic information. One of these would insist that if someone is a joint holder of a piece of genetic information, then they are entitled to it no matter what. But while we could be certain that identical twins would be trustees of the joint account, what about others? Siblings are fairly likely to be joint trustees of a given piece of genetic information, but they might not be; likewise parents, cousins, and offspring. How would we know whether someone actually is a trustee of the joint account, rather than a more-or-less possible one, without performing a test on them to ascertain whether they are? This would be onerous, and it would in any case make the joint account pointless, since they would be having the genetic test that way – and such a strategy would be open to a point (related to one made by Parker[14]) that in telling a person that she might be advised to have a genetic test, we would have given away that there is something for which she should consider having a test, and this is in itself potentially sensitive information.

However, we can avoid these problems by denying that one's interest in access to information about a genome is dependent on sharing genes. The *probability* that one shares them, on the other hand, can generate the right kind of interest, and it is at this point that we may have a reason modify the JAM. We saw in relation to the Gerry and Terry case that one of the arguments that Gerry could use against Terry's insistence on privacy is precisely that he has an interest in knowing about his own genome insofar as that might help him make decisions about his own life. But the same kind of claim could be made by relatives who do not have identical genomes: there will be some interest that Lenny and his sister Penny have in being provided with access to information that informs them about the genetic profile of their father Kenny, and potentially about each other. This interest goes beyond the extent of their joint holding in the information in question: it may encompass knowing whether they have that holding in a given piece of information to begin with. Joint holdings may explain how it is that they come to have an interest in it, and it may help explain the normative strength of that interest when it comes to deciding who may have access to what and on what terms – but it does not follow that this joint holding is the only source of the interest, or that the interest is limited by the bounds of the holding.

For example, consider *malignant hyperthermia* (MH). This is an inherited disposition to react badly – potentially fatally – to certain anaesthetic drugs. Not everyone who carries the gene will react to those anaesthetics every time they are administered. But imagine that Penny reacts badly to an anaesthetic administered during a routine operation. She recovers; her doctor, suspecting MH, refers her for a test that proves positive for the gene. Her brothers Benny and Lenny will have an interest in knowing about the casue of their sister's condition for their own sake, as will their parents Kenny and Jenny. For all, part of the relevant interest will be in being assured that they do *not* carry the gene, and therefore that part of their genome does *not* overlap with Penny's, and that they do not have a holding in this part of the joint account. Quite obviously, this interest cannot be explained as being based in a joint holding; still, it is a real interest, and it may make a normative difference. To iterate the point made a moment ago, one's interests do not arise only from a joint holding: some will arise from knowing whether one has a holding (in the relevant respect) at all. People who are trustees in a joint account will have an interest in knowing information, and to that extent it may be hard to separate the holding from the interest; but we should still be alive to the direction of travel: which obtains in its own right, and which obtains only as a product of the other.

(It might be argued that Jenny's having learned that she carries a particular gene suffices to show that Jenny and Lenny are joint holders not of a gene, but of a risk-profile, and it is this that gives Lenny a claim to access at least some information concerning his sister. But this is not what most versions of the joint account model talk about – being able to speculate in a reasonably informed way about possible genetic overlap is not the same as a true joint account, and Lenny could talk completely meaningfully about his risk profile even without being tested himself.)

This brings us to a rather crucial point: if there can be an interest in being given information that provides an insight into another person's genetic profile that does not depend on having determined a joint account, might we go further, and ditch the appeal to joint accounts as the basis and limit of access to information full stop?

This question prompts a second and a third related question: if interests determine who has what access to what information and when, what kind of interest is it that carries the weight? And how ought one to balance these interests against a putative right to privacy? Over the coming pages, I want to present a reason to think that *even if* the arguments over the previous two chapters have been unconvincing, and that *even if* one thinks that there is a robust account of privacy rights that latches on to genetic information in the right sort of way, there might still be a moral reason to share information with quite a wide range of people. Potentially, this moral reason is sufficient to outweigh the putative privacy right. But if a putative right can and should be put aside for moral reasons, what kind of right will it turn out to have been?

iv. An Obvious Exclusion

The paradigm case of the sort of party whose having access to information worries us is the insurer; if anyone is an obvious candidate for exclusion from access to information, it is the insurance agent. This is understandable: if there are goods access to which depends on being able to get insurance, and if genetic information is likely to make a difference to the affordability of insurance, then giving insurers access to it may mean some people being priced out of access to those goods. More, because genetic information strikes many people as being *deeply* about them – as referring to their very essence, unlike merely contingent information such as that concerning how much they smoke – granting too many people access to that information seems to be particularly intrusive. Jyri Liukko notes, with some plausibility, that in this respect many people's intuitive resistance to the idea that insurers ought to have any access at all to genetic information resistance flies in the face of the intuitions of many about other kinds of information:

> Traditionally it has been widely accepted that private insurers are legitimately allowed to classify and discriminate between applicants according to specific statistically relevant risk factors, particularly age, gender and health. However, in the recent debate, genetic health information is often considered to have a different moral status from that of the other classification variables. Importantly, discrimination according to all other kinds of relevant health information is deemed fair, while genetic discrimination is not. This so-called "genetic exceptionalism" [...] has been institutionalized in many European countries and in the United States through the enactment of genetic non-discrimination legislation for life and health insurance.[15]

In the United States, motivated by concerns about the use and misuse of genetic data in the workplace, and in relation to health insurance, the 2008 Genetic Information Non-Discrimination Act (GINA) set out a number of protections against discrimination based on genetic profile, and against being required to submit to genetic testing. The drafters of the Act were implicitly cognisant of genetic information's unconfinedness: for example, Title I amended the Employee Retirement Income Security Act of 1974 by adding the requirement that "[a] group health plan, and a health insurance issuer offering health insurance coverage in connection with a group health plan, shall not request or require an individual *or a family member of such individual* to undergo a genetic test".[16] Notwithstanding an important difference between requiring people to have a test, and requiring them to reveal the results of a test once taken, attitudes to genetic testing in this piece of leg-islation do nevertheless seem to be different from attitudes to other kinds of test. The idea that applicants for an insurance policy should have to provide evidence of physical health does not generate anything like as visceral a response, and it does not attract the same legislative attention.

The role of the individual in sourcing medical cover from the private sector is a characteristic that makes the US healthcare system unique in the industrialised world. One of the risks of such a system is that people may, and do, find it hard to get cover if they have *any* pre-existing conditions or predispositions. This generates a situation in which those most likely to need medical cover are likely to be those least able to access it (or at least to access it affordably). This problem would obviously crop up in respect of genetics, since a person's genome may play such a significant role determining in the medical risks they face. Hence ensuring that people have access to healthcare – which I shall take without argument to be desirable and something that a minimally-decent state would strive to guarantee – may necessitate legislative intervention to regulate what the market can ask. Still, this may not provide us with much of a reason for genetic exceptionalism, since genetic conditions may not have manifested yet and may in fact never manifest, and pre-existing somatic conditions may be just as actuarially relevant.[17] Yet while legislation such as the 1990 Americans with Disabilities Act put in place legal protections against discrimination in some circumstances, it made explicit that those protections should not be interpreted as limiting the freedom of insurers, medical providers, and so on to underwrite, classify, and administer such risks.[18] The difference between the way that genetic and non-genetic condi-tions and predispositions are handled by American law is striking.

Where access to welfare and healthcare is not so closely linked to the private sector, the need to work out how much, if any, genetic information health insurers may access may not be quite so urgent. But it would not be a non-problem: there are still things that we consider to be goods that may require insurance. One's ability to get a mortgage may depend on having a valid life-insurance policy; not being able to participate in the private insurance market may mean not being able to access the good of property-ownership. Even if property-ownership as such is not a basic good, parity of consideration when it comes to accessing the means to it is. As such, genetic information may well be relevant to many decisions that individuals make, or have the chance to make; and so there may be a moral reason to limit what information is available to at least some commercial bodies, on pain of people finding that they are priced out of certain markets based on things that they cannot control.

(Fiering notes a potential difficulty with taking the idea of things that one cannot control at face value, since lifestyle and environmental factors may well make a difference to the effect that a gene has on one's life,[19] and these are at least in principle controllable. Hence while one can do nothing about one's genes, and while there may be little that one can do about one's future health when one carries a gene for a monofactorial genetic condition with a high penetrance and no current prophylaxis, there will be other conditions that one – plausibly – could do something about. Imagine that the risk of falling ill from a genetically-related condition C can be reduced to negligible levels by some trivial and trivally-cheap intervention. But now suppose that someone refuses to make that intervention, or to have the test for the gene. In that case, it does not seem wildly implausible to think that she is in some way careless of her welfare, and that insurers may be able to say that this is the kind of thing about which they have an interest in knowing. That said, the point would still stand making that some people's genetic inheritance alters their risk profile irrespective of lifestyle or environment, and this elevated risk is a bare fact that may end up pricing some out of the market.)

In the United Kingdom, resistance to the use of genetic information has been formally recognised by the insurance industry: under some pressure from the government, it accepted a moratorium on the use of predictive genetic testing in 2005.[20] This moratorium was originally supposed to hold until 2011, but it was extended in that year: a statement from the Association of British Insurers explained that

> the results of a predictive genetic test will not affect a consumer's ability to take out any type of insurance other than life insurance over £500,000. Above this amount, insurers will not use adverse predictive genetic test results unless the test has been specifically approved by the Government. Only around 3% of all policies sold are above these limits. The only test that is approved is for Huntington's Disease.[21]

This moratorium was replaced in 2018 with an open-ended Code, which formalised the limits on the use of genetic information.[22] There is scope for the uses to which information can be put to be changed, but proposals for a change have to be agreed by the Government after a process of independent peer review.[23] Again, though, the restrictions surrounding the acquisition and use of non-genetic information are not nearly as tight as they are for genetic. This implies that the ABI has, wittingly or not, signed up to the idea that it is appropriate to protect genetic information, and to circumscribe what third parties may do with it, in a way that is not necessarily true for other kinds of information.

v. Genes and Discrimination

One very powerful reason not to fling open the doors and allow insurers access to genetic information is based on an appeal to discrimination. If people were excluded from access to some good for reasons over which they have no control, this might be deeply undesirable. There might be something of a parallel with racism here: just as it would be unjust to refuse a person insurance coverage on the basis of ethnicity, so it would be unjust to refuse her on the basis of any other fact about her that is beyond her control. The parry to this point is obvious, though: whereas racism depends on an over-estimation of the moral importance of ethnicity, a person's genetic profile *may* be of distinct interest to people like insurers, who would not necessarily be trying to get it to carry more weight than it can bear; this does create room for a moral difference.

It may be important here to try to get a bit of a tighter grip on what is going on in genetic discrimination. To treat two people differently because of their genomes is discriminatory. In the broadest sense, it is unlikely that all discrimination whatsoever is unjust. For example, the leisure centre might discriminate according to sex inasmuch as that there are some areas (changing rooms, for example) to which members of one sex don't have access. This suggests that discrimination (*qua* differential treatment) can be not only acceptable, but desirable, which indicates that merely demon-strating discrimination won't prove injustice. Nevertheless, the everyday use of the word "discrimination" has the word "unjust" as an unstated prefix. The question we have to confront as a way to getting to grips with the justifi-cation for treating genetic information in a given way as a matter of policy is one of whether an insurer charging a higher premium to someone on the basis of her DNA is necessarily an example of unjust discrimination. It ought not to be forgotten in this that discrimination – in the sense of making use of data about people to calculate a cost individuated to them, based on their risk profile – is at least in principle how private-sector insurance works. To say that insurers ought not to discriminate *at all* therefore more or less amounts to saying that private sector insurers ought to forswear something crucial to their function. And while it might well be true that a just world would not be one in which access to healthcare was decided by the availability of private-sector insurance, that's not the same as saying that a just world would make it impossible for private insurers to function. Still, if it turns out that there is even a tolerably close analogy between discrimination on the basis of something like race and discrimination on the basis of genes, we would seem to have a good moral reason to push against genetic information being shared, since the whole point of giving insurers access is to facilitate dis-crimination.

There are certain population groups in which certain genes are more common. This invites the thought that there is at least *some* connection between ethnicity and susceptibility to certain medical problems. Consider, for example, Tay-Sachs disease. Because someone needs to inherit the gene for the condition from both parents for it to manifest, this means that many people who carry the gene will be unaffected. All the same, it has an incidence of around 1 in 3,600 for Ashkenazi children, compared to 1 in 360,000 generally, and has a carrier frequency of around 1 in 30 for Ashkenazim, around ten times greater than that for the general population.[24] There are many other examples that one might dig out to show something similar. As such, we might be tempted to treat ethnicity as something of a proxy for genetic risk: if we know that a particular condition is more common among members of a certain ethnic group than among the rest of the population, we can say something about the chance that a token member of that group will manifest it. Therefore, we might expect that insurers would use ethnicity in such cases as a rough guide to risk for such conditions.

Yet this would be moving too quickly. Morally, it is likely that we would have worries about the prospect that members of certain groups might be to all intents and purposes excluded from the insurance market, and perhaps from more besides, simply because they are members of that group. Indeed, in the United States, GINA points out in its opening pages that

> many genetic conditions and disorders are associated with particular racial and ethnic groups and gender. [But b]ecause some genetic traits are most prevalent in particular groups, members of a particular group may be stigmatized or discriminated against as a result of that genetic information.[25]

This is an important point about social justice. But suppose a hard-nosed pragmatist were to argue that actuarial justice is the name of the game in private transactions, or even that social justice must take actuarial justice into account. Even then, adverting to ethnicity would be a mistake. Since it's having this or that condition, or the gene that is associated with it, that carries the statistical and actuarial weight, to look to ethnicity risk invites actuarial inaccuracy. Relying on ethnicity to gauge risk is something of a blunderbuss approach, targeting the aggregate risk presented by a whole group of people, rather than the particular risk presented by the actual individual buying the policy. If the idea is that taking ethnicity into account is desirable because it smooths out the variations between individuals, we may well wonder why we don't just smooth them out across humanity as a whole, and ditch the idea of establishing individual risk profiles. For this reason, it is plausible to expect that insurers making appeals to ethnicity in decisions about cover and premiums would quickly find themselves outcompeted by others with a more precise algorithm who could calculate premiums based on actual risk. Such insurers ought therefore to recognise a commercial reason to avoid a pricing strategy based on ethnicity even if they happened to be indifferent to the moral one. Put another way, in a properly-functioning market, ethnicity *per se* would not be used all that much as a proxy for genetic risk. It might not make all that much commercial sense, irrespective of the morality.

By contrast, it is not unreasonable to think that genetic information would be actuarially relevant in a way that ethnicity isn't: carrying a gene associated with deteriorating eyesight might be important for car insurers; a disposition towards a life-threatening illness is not irrelevant when it comes to life insurance. This is the sort of thing that an insurer – call her Perry – would want to know about. On the face of it, this will not tell us whether Perry's desire is morally legitimate; but it does give us a reason to think that even if it isn't, the reasons are different from those that apply in respect of discriminating by race. At the very least, there will be a potential commercial rationale. But this does mean that the risk that certain people might be excluded from the insurance market persists. If insurers were to use genetic profiles directly when setting premiums, it may mean that those carrying certain genes would face adverse selection problems just because their risks would be that much more certain – and, once again, we would be opening the door to people being treated differently because of contingent factors beyond their control, which might lead us to worry that there is still scope for injustice.

Yet even here, there may be cause to be sanguine. If an amoral-but-commercially-wise insurer would probably not count race as a relevant factor because it is too imprecise a measure, an analogous argument applies in respect of a person's genetic profile. Suppose that a potential client – call her Kerry – is at an elevated risk of some genetic illness. It would be unlikely that she would be absolutely uninsurable. Carrying a gene for a given condition reflects an increased probability that that condition will manifest, but this is not always a certainty. For example, a mutated BRCA-1 or BRCA-2 gene indicates a high lifetime chance of developing breast cancer: Cancer Research UK suggests that around 70% of women carrying a faulty BRCA-1 or BRCA-2 gene will develop breast cancer by the age of 80.[26] But of course, this leaves 30% who will not have shown the disease even by the age of 80 – and since 80 is a perfectly respectable age at which to die of anything at all, there is a non-zero probability that something else will kill them before any cancer had a chance to develop anyway. This is not a nice thing to think about, but it is relevant. Fate may decide that something else will kill someone. Even in relation to conditions that arise from an autosomal dominant gene, carriers of which will manifest the disease all else being equal, there is always a chance that all else will *not* be equal. A prophylactic treatment may come onto the market before the illness manifests; some carriers of the gene remain anomalously healthy. Other carriers of the gene might have the kind of lifestyle that generally shortens life anyway, in which case their carrying the gene will be neither here nor there (especially if the condition in question tends only to manifest later in life).

The point is that there is a chance, however small, that insurers will not have to pay out: they are not doomed to back a losing horse. And this means that a price can be put on the risk, and a market can exist. Whether it is a market participation in which is within the economic reach of potential clients is a different matter; and this does bring us back to the justice question. I shall address this further in a moment. But it is worth noting in the meantime that the real world does provide examples of a functioning market being able to provide insurance to notionally "uninsurable" groups. Prominent among these examples would be that of gay men, who found it more or less impossible to get insurance at the beginning of the 1980s due to concerns about HIV. However, even in the depths of the epidemic, the risk presented by HIV was still expressible in terms of probability; it could be priced, and this meant that there was a market that could be exploited.[27] The market having been opened up, HIV (and not sexuality) could – at least in principle – assume its true actuarial relevance.[28]

If Perry is a sensible insurer, she might ask that Kerry take certain health tests when her policy is up for renewal because of her genetic susceptibility; but the genetic susceptibility need not be all that much of a worry provided that Kerry's health for the duration of the policy is expected to be good. Since many policies renew annually, genetically-inherited illnesses would presumably be no different from any other condition; and it is not implausible, nor obviously unjust, that Perry would make requests for a more generalised health test. If she is selling a life-insurance policy, she might well want assurance that Kerry is displaying no irregularities in her breast tissue before agreeing a price; but this need have nothing to do with whether or not Kerry carries BRCA-1. It's the irregularities that'll worry Perry: where a price can be put on risk, a policy is sellable. Genetic exceptionalism, such as to mean that we ought to be particularly worried about the impact of genetics, is not obviously commercially warranted.

Differential treatment based on genetic inheritance is more likely to be commercially justifiable than differential treatment based on ethnicity. There is such a thing as actuarially just discrimination based on genetics, and a properly-functioning market would at least in theory find the level. But it could do so without ruling any potential buyer out in principle. That said, actuarial fairness is at most a necessary condition for fairness *sensu lato*. It might still turn out that there is no morally defensible reason to allow insurers access to genetic information, and if in practice nobody can afford the actuarially-fair premiums, it will not matter a jot that they are not excluded in principle. Neither have we yet learned much about who has the right kind of interest in accessing genetic information, since there would still be an indefinitely large number of candidates wanting to access it; but if we can show that insurers *could* make a moral case for access, and granted the assumption that insurers are among the most obviously excludable of candidates, then this would make a serious impact on the moral argument in favour of the stringent protection of putative rights to genetic privacy.

vi. Contractual Fairness

Genetic information's availability may generate difficulties when it comes to obtaining affordable insurance, and it is therefore unremarkable that many of us would prefer insurers not to have access to at least some genetic information about us. A person is rational enough in preferring that information about his susceptibility to a certain condition not be available on the grounds that his elevated risk will increase the cost of his premium; this rides on his expectation that the premium is calculated according to risk, and that that information is crucial in deciding how much of a risk he presents. Conversely, we might sometimes prefer that insurers *do* have, and make use of, information, because we think it would work to our advantage for them to do so – for example, if we could show that we definitely did *not* carry a particular gene associated with elevated morbidity or mortality, we might want that to be taken into account. But while potential clients have an interest in regulating how genetic information may be accessed with a view to how it might be used by insurers, insurers have a balancing interest of their own in being able to access it as they see fit; and that interest is most compelling in precisely those situations when potential clients would prefer that *they* maintain control over access.

Consider a simple model in which a would-be client, Kerry, is interested in buying an insurance policy from a provider, Perry. It so happens that, at least as far as English law is concerned, the general principle is that insurance contracts are considered to be *uberrimae fidei* – of the utmost good faith. This means that if relevant information is not disclosed, that may be enough for one party to treat the contract as though it never existed. Moreover,

> the proposer's opinion as to the materiality of non-disclosed facts is irrelevant even though they may well have acted in good faith. It is the law that a man may act in perfect good faith within the ordinary meaning of the phrase, yet still be held not to have acted in the utmost good faith in the legal sense.[29]

This would imply that both parties to an insurance contract should be able to access pertinent information, on pain of that contract being considered void; and it is not beyond the realms of possibility that genetic information about Kerry would be pertinent to at least some policies. Insurers may choose to forswear genetic information (as *per* the ABI's moratorium on its use); all the same, an agent's right to enter into a contract based on the fullest possible information is compatible with that agent issuing a self-denying ordinance on the matter. And while law is a poor guide to ethics, or to what law should be, the moral principle that this norm reflects seems sound enough.

A market functions best when all parties can negotiate the price for a good or service based on perfect knowledge, or knowledge that is at the very least as good as possible when perfection sets too high a standard.

However, each party also has an interest in there being an imperfection in the market, provided that it favours them. Each will be trying to get the best possible deal for themselves, and controlling information will be part of the strategy. In our example, Kerry will want to minimise the cost of a policy, and therefore has a reason to withhold information if that will help her realise her aim; Perry will want to minimise the costs potentially incurred if a claim is made, and therefore has a reason to want access to that information. It would be unfair for Perry to add clauses to the contract without telling Kerry, because Kerry has an interest in access to information about her contract and the likelihood that it will pay out. Roughly the same thing might be said on behalf of the Perry: she has an interest based in fairness in knowing what risks Kerry faces – and indirectly what she will face herself – so that a fair price can be put on them.[30]

How far does Perry's interest go? Is it in any way bankable against Kerry, so that she has an obligation of any sort to volunteer information irrespective of her desires and claims to privacy rights? My argument so far has been that entitlements to restrict access are more eroded the closer the blood relationship. This tells us little about Kerry and Perry. If Kerry has a right to genetic privacy, this may be the kind of thing that she could use to prevent Perry accessing information about her genetic profile. But I shall argue over the coming pages that Perry might have a morally weighty claim to access information about Kerry. As such, intuitions about Kerry's rights to privacy may take a knock.

vii. Relevant Persons' Relevant Interests

It is worth spending a moment to clarify on whose behalf Perry is speaking.

Insurers are firms, and so we might wonder whether firms have interests in their own right, or interests of the kind morally weighty enough to yield anything like at least a *prima facie* entitlement to genetic information. One question might concern whether a firm is ontologically the kind of thing that can have interests in the first place. Even if it is, this leaves open the further question of whether something's having interests of the right sort would depend on whether it is a person in more than the legal sense, or sentient, or something like that. If a firm is not a "thing", or if it is not the sort of thing to which interests can attach, Kerry will be much more likely to be entitled to keep her genetic information private.

But, actually, these questions are irrelevant to the current inquiry, for reasons that I'll begin to explain in the next paragraph. And even if such questions were relevant, we would not have to worry too much about the answer, because even if a firm can't have interests of its own, we can still say that it channels the interests if others who do have interests in their own right. The clients of Perry's company have interests; and there is no reason to suppose that we cannot talk about the firm's interests as a proxy for them. This will be an important component of the argument in a little while.

To see why we don't have to worry too much about the ontology of insurance companies, we can simplify matters by treating Perry as a private individual, assuming that whatever interests Perry has ought to be indicative of the interests that firms have *tout court*. So imagine that Kerry is reluctant to buy an insurance policy from a corporation, but that Perry is a wealthy and statistically savvy acquaintance who happens also to be a cautious but willing gambler, and offers to cover Kerry's liabilities in the event of misfortune. In return, Kerry will pay Perry a small amount, calculated according to the size of the liability and the chance that Perry will have to pay out. In this setup, Perry would have a reasonable moral claim to relevant information, based in her interest in knowing the terms upon which she and Kerry are to enter into their agreement. Granted that there are times when genetic information might be relevant, there's a perfectly workaday way of arguing that not to share it would not be fair.

But if Kerry has an obligation in respect of one rich friend, then why not the same obligation in respect of two less-rich (but cumulatively rich-enough) friends? Or three? Or a few hundred? Why not, in short, a firm in a more conventional sense? Maybe what makes the difference is that Kerry can be acquainted with a certain number of specific people, but cannot have the same kind of social ties to a group of people arranged into, or represented by, a commercial organisation. Social acquaintance is not quite the same as friendship proper, but it is perhaps friendship *in embryo*, or it may be something to which we would want to add the label "special purpose friendship"[31]; and it is not unreasonable to entertain the possibility that we have moral ties to identifiable individuals whom we know in a way that we do not have to complete strangers, considered singly or *en bloc* – and Kerry and Perry presumably know each other reasonably well, since their arrangement does rely on trust. Social bonds are certainly morally important. However, my obligation to be honest with friends and acquaintances about relevant information does not seem to be based entirely on an appeal to the moral importance of friendship, and whatever obligations we have specifically to friends, honesty is not one of them: we owe that to everyone. Honesty is, of course, not the same as candour, and it may be a bit much to expect Kerry to *offer* information to Perry. Still, it would also be implausible to suppose that Perry might not ask for it, and that if she were to ask for it, she would not have a reasonable expectation of a full and truthful answer. Besides, a lack of candour may potentially amount to a kind of dishonesty should it predictably lead to others inferring a distorted view of the relevant facts. Alternatively, we may be heading from the realm of the private to the realm of the secret; and even if there is a right to privacy, it does not follow that things we say about that would translate to things we would say about keeping secrets from an interested party. Remember, after all, that a characteristic of secrets is that there are reasons to tell them.

Perhaps more importantly, there are plenty of circumstances in which we do attribute to organisations such as firms something like the moral status that we recognise in individuals. We assign responsibilities to firms, some-times retrospectively, such as when we seek to apply a sanction for their having done things that we would have preferred them not to have done (perhaps, for the sake of the argument, when they have made use of genetic data in a way we think they ought not), and sometimes prospectively, such as when it comes to deciding that they should behave in certain ways (as when we say that, henceforward, they should foreswear the use of genetic data when it comes to calculating insurance premiums).[32] It is possible that firms could have liabilities and obligations, but no corresponding rights or enti-tlements; but there is no clear way to make sense of the supposition that there is something in the *nature* of the firm that would make it capable of having liabilities and obligations but not rights or entitlements. And so, for as long as we are willing to say that firms could have liabilities and obliga-tions, we cannot dismiss as a matter of principle the idea that they could have entitlements. The nature, number, and extent of those entitlements may be an open question; but that does not cast doubt on whether they could be held at all. We accept happily enough that corporations have *some* moral sub-stance; and if they are substantial enough to have responsibilities, it is not obvious why they cannot in principle be substantial enough to have some-thing at least resembling entitlements.

Some will still want to deny that there is enough of a moral similarity between firms and people to be able to say that firms can be thought of as rights-holders. Yet the idea of the firm can serve as a convenient shorthand for other things and people. So even if one rejects the notion of a corporate moral status comparable to persons', a firm can still be characterised as a proxy for a group of other stakeholders. In the case of an insurance company, those stakeholders will be the owners or shareholders, and the other pol-icyholders, so that agreements with companies are properly to be seen as agreements with the stakeholders in those companies at one remove. *Qua* stakeholders, there is a fairness claim to be made here about their access to information: they might well have a reasonable interest in the firm having information accessible, even if that firm doesn't have any rights or interests of its own. And along these lines it would be *prima facie* plausible for share-holders to complain that they were being unfairly expected to carry the cost of an agreement between Kerry and Perry entered into on incomplete information: again, if Kerry were prevented from knowing some detail about the policy she was about to sign, we might well think that this situation would demand remedy, and it's hard to see why the same considerations wouldn't apply in the other direction.

And this helps us see a related consideration: that among those stake-holders represented by Perry will be any number of policyholders, each of whose individual premium helps cover the cost of successful claims made by other policyholders. An insurer's ability to pay out to a claimant will depend on the size of the pot from which it is able to draw. If we allow individual policyholders to withhold relevant information, the insurer will know this, and will act accordingly. In practice, this means that it will have a reason to inflate premiums to a touch above the level dictated by apparent risk and actuarial fairness in order to take account of the fact that apparent and real risk will differ. But this, in turn, means that those whose genetic profiles do *not* demonstrate a higher risk will be paying over the odds – which seems to be unfair. To that extent, as the representative of those other extant policyholders who would be subsidising Kerry's policy, Perry would seem to have a defensible moral reason to expect that she would be forthcoming with relevant genetic information. Hence it seems reasonable to think that Perry could ask Kerry for relevant information, potentially including genetic information, and could expect a truthful response; and this is because the other policyholders, whose premiums help fund any payout that any other policyholder receives, carry the cost of Kerry's policy. Likewise, Kerry would have a moral reason based in fairness and a regard for the interests of other stakeholders to reveal information that one might reasonably think relevant.[33]

But this being the case, we might wonder what had happened to her supposed right to privacy. If there is information that one has a moral reason to bring, or to allow to be brought, into the interpersonal domain, then in what sense is that compatible with a right keep it out of that domain? Kerry would still be able to assert that she had a defensible moral *reason* not to de-privatise the information; but not all reasons are rights. Hence to jump directly from asserting a reason to keep information private to asserting a right to keep it private (that is, to the claim that Perry had no bankable entitlement to the information) is no small thing. And this is because a right to privacy would be precisely what is contested.

Note that this does not come close to saying that Perry, on behalf of the people she represents, has any kind of entitlement to access *all* information about Kerry. There is a relevance criterion to satisfy. Nevertheless, there may be times when other people have perfectly plausible moral reasons to request information that we might otherwise think private, and when we ought (for reasons of fairness) to accede to those requests. And some of this information may be genetic.

viii. Profit and Profiteering

Is any of this modified by the fact that firms and their shareholders are motivated by profit? If the process of negotiating a premium is effectively a game of strategy in which insurers look to maximise what they can charge and minimise what they pay out, it does not invite much in the way of generosity from those firms: the ad-man's insistence that insurance compa-nies really care about their clients is reassuring, but it is patently false. We might think that there is not all that much reason to make life easy for firms that are motivated by self-interest; disclosure, seen through this prism, may not seem all that attractive. However, there's an easy *tu quoque* response to this, since customers will also be looking to minimise what they are charged and maximise what they are paid. The reason why a person like Kerry would *not* want to share genetic information with an insurer is – presumably – so that she can ensure a favourable price for herself. In efect, she is seeking to maximise her own profit. The motivating attitude is the same for companies as it is for clients; if it's wrong for Perry and her colleagues to seek to maximise benefit and minimise outlay for themselves, then the same would seem to apply to Kerry.

Maybe we should worry not so much about profit, as about *profiteering*: not so much that firms are looking to make the outcome as good as possible for themselves, as that they are doing so from a point of unfair advantage and capitalising on Kerry's presumed vulnerability. Insurance cover is a necessity for many quite everyday things; to some extent, Perry and her boardroom colleagues may already have potential customers over the proverbial barrel. This is compounded by the fact that insurance companies have the actuarial muscle to name their price, which means that there is a clear power differential between individuals and firms. Even in the simplified version of the example in which Perry is an individual, she possesses unusual insight into risk, and Kerry is unlikely to be able to challenge the price she is quoted or to negotiate as an equal. This inequality is amplified in the relationship of individuals to firms, which have massive actuarial resources at their disposal. It is always for them to propose a price to Kerry to take or leave, rather than *vice versa*. There is, accordingly, a concern about a kind of epistemic injustice that we may be inclined to raise here.

The term "epistemic injustice" here uses, but slightly reworks, a term coined by Miranda Fricker. Fricker is largely concerned with epistemic injustice in the form of what she calls "testimonial injustice", by which "prejudice on the hearer's part causes him to give the speaker less credibility than he would otherwise have given",[34] and in which "someone is wronged in their capacity as a giver of knowledge".[35] One example of this would be a situation in which a person who ought to be believed on some matter has her expertise discounted: she suffers from a credibility deficit because of who she is, or some fact about her, rather than because of any lack of knowledge. But there is more to it than simply not receiving a fair share of the good of credibility, since "this would fail to capture the distinctive respect in which the speaker is wronged". Rather, the injustice here is, Fricker suggests, "a kind of injustice in which someone is wronged specifically in her capacity as a knower".[36] And there is more than one way in which a person may be the subject of epistemic injustice: Fricker herself supplements her talk of testimonial injustice by talking of "hermeneutical injustice", which arises "when a gap in collective interpretive resources puts someone at an unfair disadvantage when it comes to making sense of their social experiences".[37] There being more than one kind of epistemic injustice is important, since it allows us to say that it may arise in the Kerry and Perry case. Kerry is unable to negotiate as an equal because the knowledge that she would need to do so is likely to be beyond her, as it would be beyond any plausible person. As such, she is at risk of being taken for a ride, and would, in effect, be vulnerable to willingly entering into a contract that is unjust. This is clearly related to hermeneutic injustice, but it is not quite the same; it is not so much that the conceptual framework to articulate a wrong does not exist, so much as that the whole field of play is tipped against her. Kerry cannot engage with Perry freely as an equal. (This concern is not quite the same as Rawlsian worries about "background justice" being distorted by "oligopolistic configurations of accumulations that succeed in maintaining unjustified inequalities and restrictions on fair opportunity",[38] but it is clearly in the same family.) The routinisation of disclosure about things such as genetic information may be felt to leave people like Kerry prey to profiteering, because they will have simply no idea about what a just settlement or even negotiation would look like.

Would the disclosure of information really allow profiteering? We should note that the nature of the relationship between information and profit in a free market means that the charge of profiteering does not always stick. One of the features that characterises a perfect free market is that both buyers and sellers have full information, which implies full disclosure and knowledge of risk profiles. In such a market, profits would tend towards zero, because, if an insurer is making a £5 profit from Kerry, a rival will know it, and be incentivised to enter the market and offer a similar policy at a lower price. This rival will make a smaller profit – £4, say – but since he gets the business, this doesn't matter, since it'll be £4 more than he would have made. On the Micawberish principle that all that matters for there to be an incentive to enter the market is that *some* profit can be made, the cycle can continue until the expected profit reaches zero. In a perfect market – that is to say, one in which Kerry can shop around between several sellers – there is no room for profiteering because there's very nearly no room for profit. So long as Kerry knows that there are several competing suppliers, she will be able to use that knowledge to optimise her position in the market. If we have faith in the idea that a properly-functioning market is a guard against the injustice represented by profiteering, the cost of that is privacy and the entitlement to withhold information as we see fit.

All of this may be true, but it will be irrelevant when, as in the real world, markets do not operate perfectly. Appealing to the desirability of a free flow of information is mere pabulum if only one of the parties can possibly be expected to do anything useful with it: insurance markets are doomed to be imperfect in that sense. On the other hand, the defender of the free market may still be able to say that it is not necessary for Kerry to be the epistemic match of Perry. All that is necessary is that there is a range of potential insurance brokers, each of whom is as epistemically well-prepared as the others, and each of whom wants to woo Kerry. So long as that condition is satisfied, our concerns about profiteering ought to be soothed, because each potential seller will be trying to steal a march on the others, and this cannot help but to work in Kerry's favour.

I am no more persuaded of the existence of perfect (or even as-good-as-possible) markets than I am of fairies. But what matters *at this stage of the argument* is simply that Kerry's genetic information being made available to Perry is not *necessarily* going to result in Kerry's exploitation. All the same, it would be naïve to suppose that, because information flows freely in a perfect market, making Kerry's genetic information freely available is a desirable step towards perfecting the market. Some steps towards a perfected market may, when taken on their own, actually make things worse for at least one participant, and so the anti-profiteering argument for liberal flows of genetic information is compelling only in ideal, or near-ideal, situations. And because the world and its markets are imperfect, we may conclude that sharing information will be much more likely to benefit one party than the other, and that the party that benefits more will be the more powerful one; and we may deduce that the more powerful party in the formation of most insurance contracts is the insurance company. And we might have precious little sympathy for the kind of people who own insurance companies, and lose no sleep over the idea that they might prefer that information be shared.

The conclusion at this point may run along the lines that, absent a perfect market, there are good reasons to suppose that a client such as Kerry might legitimately impose restrictions on what Perry could know, and that her reasons for restricting access would count against her reasons to disclose. Nevertheless, it is not clear that "This information is private" would imply a right of privacy, or that it would count in itself as a reason not to disclose. If we are satisfied that Perry has a claim to access certain information about Kerry for the sake of maintaining fairness – fairness in pricing, and fairness to all relevant stakeholders – then for Kerry to insist that she has an *ab initio* right to privacy that counts against such access would seem to commit her to the view that a right to privacy is a right that might militate against fairness. Put another way, if we think that fairness could be furthered by disclosure, then for Kerry to stand on a putative right to maintain privacy would appear to be for her to endorse unfairness as a matter of right, which is odd.

The other option would be to say that there were competing rights in play, such as rights to privacy, and to fairness. But all that would do would be to push the question back a stage: if there are competing rights, then simply asserting a right cannot be enough to settle a dispute about what should be done: we would have to try to say which right prevailed on this occasion. But this would give the game away: the "right to ..." part of each party's claim would cancel out. If we can talk about one such claim being the more powerful and say why it is more powerful, then it is that rather than the rights claim that makes the moral difference.

A concern for fairness would mean that we ought to consider whether information that would otherwise be hidden from the interpersonal domain perhaps ought to be brought into that domain at least on some occasions.

Looking at matters this way would allow us to acknowledge Kerry's interests in keeping the information to herself; but those interests would be moral reasons among others, with a "right" to privacy assigned on the basis of which interests prevail in this context. If sharing the information would mean that Kerry is treated as a non-equal, or excluded from some basic good, then her interests in maintaining privacy may win out. But if we decide that, all things considered, she ought to share the information, then we are *pro tanto* saying that she has no right not to – that is implicit in *ought* statements. This amounts to saying that she has no right to keep information out of the interpersonal domain, and that she therefore cannot appeal to a right to genetic privacy, at least in this case. By the same token, if we decide that the proper moral consideration of things forces the conclusion that she may deny Perry access to a given piece of genetic information, her "right" is a kind of epiphenomenon: a way of describing our conclusion that she need not share the information after all. What matters is that there may be times when, for moral reasons, one ought to allow others access to information, even if that information is potentially sensitive. And if that is the case, then a "right to privacy" looks to be a fairly notional sort of thing.

ix. Insurance and Taboo?

If we are going to talk about privacy in respect of information, then at least one person – probably the referent – must be able to access it. If the referent cannot access it, we are talking about a secret or a taboo. And something similar can be said in respect of the use of that information. A person may want others not to be able to access information about her based on a concern that it would be put to use, possibly detrimentally; but this is compatible with thinking that an autonomous agent would be entitled to make use of information as she sees fit. To deny that also seems to make private information taboo. This does not seem like all that attractive a picture. As such, if Kerry has a *right* to privacy in respect of genetic information (and certainly if this right is a facet of informational privilege), then we would expect her to be able to access information about herself, and potentially to put it to use.

The flipside of the thought that insurers have a reason to pursue disclosure is that clients have reasons not to disclose both because of the possible consequences of disclosure, and because of a common-or-garden appeal to autonomy in being able to decide for ourselves whether and under what circumstances we should disclose potentially sensitive information. A universalisation of that principle would indicate that *any* agent should have the same interests. And, indeed, we may have a higher-order interest in living in the kind of society in which people can choose to do with information that concerns them as they please.

But people can have conflicting interests, and they can have interests that they do not know they have. In fact, Kerry has an interest in people *not* being able to share or withhold information as they see fit. We have seen the seeds of why this is already: she, as a policyholder, will have a stake in other policyholders being candid about their risks. But there is slightly more to things than that.

Allow that Kerry knows the details of her genome, and can make at least an educated guess about her risk of being diagnosed with a given life-threatening condition. On the presumption that the more likely it is and the sooner it is that something undesirable is to happen the more rational it is to insure against it, we can deduce that if she knows herself to be at low risk, she will be correspondingly less likely to insure against it, having better things to do with her money. But this means that allowing people to use information they have about themselves to decide whether to buy insurance, and what kind of insurance to buy, will tend to skew the market: there will be an unrealistically high proportion of high-risk people buying. This will force up prices, because the aggregate risk faced by insurers will be that much higher, with a lower number of low-risk policyholders whose premiums ensure the solvency of any pot from which payouts would be drawn. Those at high risk would therefore be forced to pay more than they would have otherwise. As Andrew McGee notes,

> widespread genetic testing has the potential to undermine the life assurance industry. At present the industry works on the basis that those who live long will by their premiums pay for those who die young, all parties taking a gamble on their life expectancy when the policy is taken out. If the element of gamble is significantly reduced, then it may be that those with a long life expectancy will be less inclined to insure, leaving only a pool of poorer risks, whose premiums will have to increase to a point where insurance may be too expensive for them. On this theory the industry would do well to discourage the practice of genetic testing.[39]

Whereas in one sense the industry, as a network of stakeholders – some shareholders, some policyholders – each of whom has a set of *prima facie* morally-defensible interests, may have an interest in genetic information being known so that it can be disclosed and used, it may have another interest in its not being.

As it happens, when Hoy and Witt modelled what would happen if proposers were allowed to know their own genetic risk but keep that information from insurers, they concluded that

> the size of adverse selection costs generated by a regulation prohibiting insurers from using genetic test results for the BRCA1/2 genes would probably be very modest in most circumstances. Thus, equity and privacy arguments that favor such regulation would not pale in comparison.

Yet, they continue,

> for some higher-risk family background types, if women in sufficient numbers obtain genetic tests, then adverse selection costs from such regulation could be substantial. This points to the possibility that as genetic information in society grows, there may come a point when genetic privacy may not be desirable.[40]

If people could choose to guard their privacy or share information, this may result in some people paying more for insurance. This effect could be in line with actuarial fairness.[41] But there are possible situations in which allowing the proposer but not the insurer to know her genetic profile may be the worst arrangement in terms of fairness more widely conceived.

On the assumption that the principles that motivate Kerry's preferences ought to be equally applicable to all, the situation would appear to be that, notwithstanding her fairness-based reason to allow Perry to access (certain) information about her genetic profile that sits alongside her rational self-interest in keeping the information private, Kerry might well also prefer that Perry has access to the same information from others: she has a reason to deny that their claims to privacy rights suffice to prevent access to information. But she would thereby either sacrifice her own putative right to privacy on the altar of actuarial fairness, or have to come up with a way for the rules that apply to others not to apply to her.

Saying that insurers may not make use of (certain) genetic information when calculating a premium would certainly help ensure that insurance was accessible to those with elevated dispositions to certain conditions; and though it would elevate the cost of everyone's premium, so long as the pool was big enough, the marginal difference may well be small – and a price worth paying for the sake of fairness. However, this strategy may overshoot, since it says nothing about the ability of potential clients to make decisions about whether to buy insurance. Here, the problem is that for Kerry to have a meaningful right to privacy in respect of her genome implies that she would have access to that information herself, and (assuming that the principles underpinning what she may and may not do are universal) everyone else would have access to theirs. But any potential buyer with access to this kind of information will be able to use it to make strategic decisions about whether to seek insurance at all. If Gerry learns that he has no genetic timebombs ticking away, this will inform his decisions about the best use he can make of his money: insurance might be the worst. The net effect will be that there will be a proportionate relationship between the desire of Perry's clients for insurance, and the risks that they face – which means that Kerry may still be facing very high premiums, since the funds required to cover payments to those who *do* buy a policy will have to come from somewhere. This situation could be avoided if potential clients were not able to use what they know about their own genomes to inform their decisions about buying insurance – but that is implausible: nobody could be required to bracket such knowledge. And so the next best alternative would be to say that, actually, this counts as a reason to think that people ought to remain in ignorance about their own genomes. But this would shift genetic information from the private to the taboo.

When push comes to shove, then, a market for private insurance in a world in which we think that there is a right to genetic privacy would mean that we have to settle on one horn of a dilemma: either we opt for something that is suboptimal in terms of fairness, or we admit that insurers may have a legitimate claim to at least some genetic information. There is an arguable case to share at least some genetic information at least some of the time; and if that argument ever prevails – especially in respect of an organisation like an insurance company – then the idea that there is a thoroughgoing right to genetic privacy such as could generate a veto to access goes by the board. And once we have accepted that this strong view of genetic privacy rights is untenable, then we have to accept that we are simply talking about moral reasons to maintain privacy in balance with moral reasons to allow access. As indicated above, we can have the important moral debates about who should have access to what information and on what terms, without there being much of a place for the language of rights at all.

An important consideration in all of this would be whether Kerry has options to access basic goods without private insurance. If access to even basic healthcare depends on private insurance, the risks that she faces by virtue of being priced out of the market would be potentially great. (In this context, when Evans *et al* suggest that "the more clinically useful the test, the more it should be readily accessible to health care providers",[42] it is slightly puzzling that they pay no heed to the implications that this may have for accessibility: their implicit assumption seems to be that the *uberimma fides* of the private insurance contract is the only thing that matters.[43]) But if access to at least basic healthcare is underwritten by the state, then any inaccessibility of private health insurance would represent less of a threat. Such a society is preferable to its *laissez-faire* alternative. Moreover, once the potential costs of covering high-risk individuals is covered by the public sector, then this is likely to make a market for private insurance optional, and thereby focused on elective medicine – and so it would be less affected by genetic risk, and correspondingly that much more accessible to everyone. Meanwhile, a public-sector health system would be so big as to make the risks that it carries nugatory, and the nugatory burden that Kerry presents to everyone else would be amenable to justification by means of an appeal to desirable characteristics such as solidarity.[44] I shall talk more about solidarity as a moral principle later; but a point that presents itself here is that, since genomes are shared between persons anyway, this should right from the start have tipped us off that a wholly individualistic approach to how to think about them and their role in social policy would set us off on the wrong foot. It would certainly be fallacious to leap directly from "We share our genes with other people" to "Therefore there should be a mandatory public health sector". However, thinking clearly about the unconfinedness of genetic information, and the shared nature of genes, forces us to abandon much that we might otherwise take for granted in respect of the individual as the sovereign locus of moral concern, and so sits nicely with a more communitarian account of healthcare provision.

In a like manner, a society with decent social housing and public transport, or which was willing and able to cross-subsidise excess risk that any one person might represent in comparison to the average within the population, would be one in which being priced out of private insurance would be less likely to matter. In such cases, the argument from fairness for allowing Perry access to genetic information about Kerry would be that much stronger.

(When it comes to things like eligibility for a mortgage, which may depend on being able to get insurance, we need to consider whether it is home-ownership that is a basic good, or simply housing. An important factor here is that homeownership is serves as a store of wealth that can be passed down the generations. The descendants of someone who cannot get a mortgage may therefore have worse start in life than the descendants of someone who can: genetic inheritance may stymie testamentary inheritance. However, I do not think that we could plausibly say that inherited wealth is a basic good. What we could much more plausibly say is that a world is less just when inherited wealth matters to a person's opportunities and decisions. I shall leave this slight digression hanging. Readers may take or leave it as they will.[45])

To be clear: in none of this am I saying that insurers really do have an entitlement to genetic information: each of the points I have raised may be defeated. But what matters is that their having access is arguable, and simply saying that they may not access it because of an *ab initio* right to privacy is taking an awful lot for granted. Equally, if we are treating such a right as a *datum* of moral debate, then it will come up against other plausible claims to rights of access, in which case their being rights will prove to be of no consequence: we would still have to decide which right is the more powerful, and *qua* right each would cancel out. The moral decision would be made elsewhere; and so it would be more efficient to go directly to that point and let the "rights" part sort itself out later.

x. Other Rights of Access

Whatever conceptual problems there may be with the idea of rights to genetic privacy, there may be moral reasons not to stand on those rights. There are moral reasons not to stand on *any* rights that we may have – it is sometimes honourable to relinquish them. But in the normal run of things, if we have the right to φ, then we will not have wronged anyone else by φ-ing; they have no entitlement to our not φ-ing. Yet there may be circumstances in which agents can claim that they are entitled to access at least some genetic information about others. And if we are satisfied that someone is entitled to access genetic information, then for the referent to insist that they oughtn't because doing so would violate a right of that referent is not going to be definitive, and may suggest an *ignoratio elenchi* fallacy. The referent's interests in maintaining privacy may be a factor in deciding whether another party is entitled to access; but it is not obvious that the argument must stop there. A claimed right to privacy is not necessarily the overriding moral consideration. It will have to fight its corner, taking into account other considerations such as fairness – and not just fairness.

What goes for insurance goes for other contexts. For example, law enforcement agencies may very well have reasons to access banks of genetic information when trying to solve a crime: matching a genetic profile from the crime scene with a sample held somewhere would be very useful for the prosecution and the defence, since it could help rule a suspect in or out. In a like manner, similar techniques (which de Groot *et al* have dubbed "investigative genetic genealogy"[46] (IGG)) could help identify sex-tourists who have fathered children, in the hope that they could be made to provide financial support to those children. Assuming this information was not misused, there would seem to be a moral good that could be furthered by discounting claims about privacy, and so a reason to consider such a discount. This does not mean that that the doors should be flung open and access granted unquestioningly. Perry's claim against Kerry to access information about her genome does not mean that Perry has a claim to access *all* the information about Kerry's genome: we might limit things, so that Perry would be entitled to know about the presence or absence of certain markers, for the sake of certain kinds of policy. In a similar fashion, allowing law-enforcement agencies access to genetic information in some circumstances does not mean that they would be permitted to access all genetic information, or to carry out a trawl of databases themselves. (de Groot *et al* provide a detailed account of the differences between information gleaned from DtC tests, and more "traditional" ways in which genetic information has been used forensically.) Nevertheless, stored genetic information has proven itself to be useful in hunting down certain criminals, and the case of the "Golden State Killer" is a good example of this.

The Golden State Killer was the epithet given to the perpetrator of a string of murders, rapes, and burglaries carried out across California in the 1970s and 1980s. It was not until 2020 that one Joseph James DeAngelo was convicted of them. The conviction was made possible by running DNA gathered at the scene though an open-source genetic databank of 1.4 million profiles called GEDmatch. GEDmatch presents itself as a genealogy service: in its own words,

> GEDmatch is a free DNA comparison and analysis website for people who have tested their autosomal DNA using a direct-to-consumer genetic testing company, such as 23andMe, or have a custom file from

other sources. Testers download their DNA data file from the testing company, and then upload it to GEDmatch. GEDmatch processes the file, adds it to a genealogical database, and provides applications for matching and further analysis.[47]

By comparing crime-scene samples with the records uploaded voluntarily to GEDmatch, investigators were able to generate a list of matches, which they could then work through in the hope of homing in on the perpetrator:

> Through familial searching on GEDmatch, investigators identified distant relatives of DeAngelo – including family members directly related to his great-great-great-great grandfather dating back to the 1800s. Based on this information, investigators built about 25 family trees. The tree that eventually linked to the Golden State Killer alone contained approximately 1000 people. Over the course of a few months, investigators used other clues like age, sex and place of residence to rule out suspects populating these trees, eliminating suspects one by one until only DeAngelo remained.[48]

The investigation of the case relied on third parties being given access to, and using, genetic information, apparently without the referents being informed. And this clearly raises questions about the propriety of such access. Worries about the implications for privacy were articulated in the media,[49] and have found voice across the academic literature as well.[50] Obviously, if storers of genetic information make it clear in the terms of service that volunteers' information may be shared, then there would be fewer grounds for complaint; and others have suggested (perhaps with a little naïvety) that privacy can be maintained because IGG as it stands does not rely on disclosing the raw data of genetic profiles, and because there is a commercial incentive to ensure that this remains the case.[51] But even if we agree that law-enforcement agencies having access to such information would be a violation of users' privacy, it would remain to be seen whether such access would be something we would want to forbid, all things considered. It is not obvious that it would. Sometimes, there could be a morally-defensible public good served by bringing information into the interpersonal domain. And – as with the insurance example – this raises a question: if we think that on certain occasions it would be permissible for the information to be accessed regardless of the referents' assent, what work is being done by the term "right to privacy" in discussions? Privacy is an important consideration when assessing permissibility; but since whether privacy is something that comes out on top of other considerations is the matter that is up for debate, calling it a *right* from the get-go is loading the dice.

Such a loading is entirely in keeping with what I called the "standard model" of bioethics, and the frequently autonomy-heavy application of the "Georgetown mantra"; but since the unconfined nature of genetic information chips away at the standard model anyway, to rely on that model to decide what to do with genetic information is not obviously the best possible approach.

I would iterate that willingness to grant access in some circumstances is not a willingness to grant access in all; neither is it saying that police forces may permissibly carry out a trawl whenever they feel like it. There would have to be an articulable reason, the power of which is open to scrutiny and moral evaluation. And care ought to be taken to ensure that the presumption of innocence without proof of guilt is not reversed so that everyone is presumed to be a legitimate suspect unless there is proof that they are not. In this light, it is notable that when Guerrini *et al* talk about the hunt for the Golden State Killer, they mention that "officers queried the genetic data of individuals who had done nothing to raise police suspicions".[52] Tacit in this is a rejection of the saw that if one has nothing to hide, one has nothing to fear, the obvious rejoinder to which is that being always subject to intrusion is itself something to fear. These are reasons for the police *not* to expect blanket access, or perhaps even access at all; they are also reasons that count against a universal databank.[53] Still, to have a reason to think that p or that *not-q* is not to show that p or *not-q* obtain. Whether third parties such as law-enforcement agencies have a convincing claim to be able to access genetic information will be arguable, and it is not implausible to suppose that there is a good that would be served by allowing it – in which case, again, a "right" to genetic privacy would be formalistic at most.

Or consider ABC, the English case brought by the daughter (ABC) of a man (XX) found to have Huntington's disease. Her claim was that she ought to have been informed of this fact about her father, not least because it impinged on her and on her reproductive decisionmaking. Much of the commentary on the case has treated it as representing a problem about confidentiality; whether it really is a matter of confidentiality, privacy, or secrecy is less important to me here than is the idea that, one way or another, he had assumed that certain things that his carers knew about him and his genome were not to be shared with his daughter; and the information was not intended to be accessible to her. Now, ABC could still have had a genetic test, and in doing so she would have learned something about her father. As such, had the information about his condition not been revealed, her rights to know about herself would not have been eroded.

But while it is true that in principle anybody could find a willing medic and book a Huntington's test for themselves, most of us do not; most of us do not think we are at particular risk from the illness. As such, XX's carers did have *a reason* to tip off ABC about her risk. Whether that was enough of a reason to mean that they ought to have told her is a further question; but an assertion made on XX's behalf that they ought not to have *just because* it would violate his rights obscures what is morally difficult about cases like this by leading us to think that there was not really a problem to solve to begin with. If "I have a right that you not φ" is supposed to mean "You must not φ", then it would not obviously have been improper for the carers to answer along the lines that that was precisely what was up for debate. If it is supposed to mean something softer, along the lines that "You have a moral reason not to φ, based at least in part my interests and my preference that you not φ", they would have been able to agree with this wholeheartedly, but still to have thought that there were counter-vailing reasons for φ-ing. And perhaps the conclusion to be drawn would have depended on the nature of the illness in question. As indicated when I considered Gerry and Terry in chapter 3, the importance of keeping information under wraps may be a function of what can be done with that information if it is shared. The penetrance of a given gene, the availability of prophylaxis, the chance that a carrier will become ill in the near future, the carrier's reproductive plans, and so on would all be relevant considerations when it comes to deciding what kind of entitlement she would have to be told that getting a test might be a good idea. And in all these cases, for the primary referent of the information to insist that the only relevant consideration is his preference for information not to be shared would be much too simple a way of looking at matters.

XX's privacy was violated: information that would not by default have been available to ABC was provided to her. But a violation of privacy is not a violation of a *right* to privacy, and we cannot infer the latter from the former. Not all violations of privacy are necessarily wrongful: a claimed privacy right may lose out in comparison to other claims. As suggested in chapter 2, there may be times when a person who has access to information to which she ought not to have access may have a responsibility to do what she can to pretend to herself that she does know what she does in fact know. If the information shared in ABC had had to do with a brain injury rather than anything genetic, ABC perhaps ought to have tried to suppress what she learned, however much of a charade that would have been in practice. But in the actual ABC case, the information shared was in some degree about ABC herself, since her genome was half derived from her father: the stake that she had in the information was qualitatively different from the stake that she would have had in "regular", confined, medical information. The onus on her to try to forget it would therefore not have been as pressing. The demands that her father's privacy made on her would not have been the same as they would have been had that information been confined, and concerned only him. Making use of unwittingly-obtained private information when it concerns oneself is not nearly so obviously *infra dig.*

What about the duties of the medical staff? Even if there were morally powerful reasons for ABC to have been told about her risk of Huntington's, we ought not to forget that medical staff who knew about XX's diagnosis would have had a moral reason both to share, and not to share, the latter being based in considerations such as the trust that XX had presumably invested in them. Even if ABC had had a claim to the information, it would not automatically follow that XX's carers would have been the ones to furnish her with it; it is possible that (following the schema outlined in chapter 2) they ought to have seen it as secret. Again, merely taxonimising information will not tell us what we ought to do with it; but it does help to clarify the nature of the dilemma we face. I'll return to this point in chapters 7 and 8.

xi. Rights, Claims, and Parsimony

We know from the argument in previous chapters that the idea of a right to genetic privacy generates problems and paradoxes, and there is plenty of reason to suppose that we have reasons to move from an individualistic way of looking at gene-carriers to something more familial. But no matter how uncompelling we find those considerations in their own right, they would still potentially come up against something fundamental in the supposed right to privacy.

Suppose someone were to insist that there is a right to genetic privacy that stands no matter how desirable it would be to share it. And suppose that an explanation of this right would rely on some level at an interest that it serves. It is possible that there will be times when the interests in which those rights are based run up against other interests that could properly be considered rights-generating themselves, or when a supposed right to genetic privacy will run up against others' rights to be treated as equals. In these cases, it looks like we have a conflict of rights; and for each disputant to stand on those rights will reflect what Emily Postan has called "endgame inflexibility",[54] which would militate against the practical import of any rights that may be involved. (A choice theorist about rights would want to say that a right to privacy is a right inasmuch as that it articulates a duty owed to the rights-holder that the rights-holder can waive; but once we begin to ask what the basis is of that duty, we find ourselves in much the same cleft stick; whatever can be said about one set of duties could at least sometimes be said about its reflection.)

Either way, there will be times when we will have to put one of the claimed (sets of) rights to one side: even if we think that there could be a right to genetic privacy, there may be situations in which others have a plausible and compelling claim to have access to certain genetic information. Yet a putative right against a person's accessing information that nevertheless is insufficient to show that they ought not to access it is, in practice, hardly worth anything – and rights are supposed to make a practical difference. The the word "right" seems to carry little weight; the moral action takes place elsewhere.

The adherent to the idea of rights might want to intervene at this point, and say that we can save the concept of the right in situations like this by talking about *prima facie* rights. Kerry and Perry might, on reflection, both have *prima facie* rights in respect of genetic information about Kerry. But where does this get us? We would still need to provide some account of which of these conflicting *prima facie* rights would and should win out in practical decisionmaking; as such, *"prima facie"* right seems to mean little more than "the kind of thing that would be normatively compelling were there no countervailing moral considerations" – which is as much as to say that it is as yet a candidate right. But a candidate right is not a right, any more than a candidate for the Presidency of the USA is a President. Again, the moral action is elsewhere.

What remains to be seen is what the operant moral considerations are; I turn to those in the next chapter. For the time being, it is sufficient to say that, should someone claim a right to privacy in respect of genetic information and deploy it as a reason to prevent others having access, we ought to treat the claim as a statement about the desired outcome of a moral debate, rather than as a *datum* within that debate. If there is no countervailing statement, the claim will go through on the Newtonian principle that things that meet no resistance will keep on moving; we will be entitled to say that the claimant does have a right to privacy after all. The same applies if there are countervailing statements that are weaker. But sometimes, the countervailing statement will have a good deal of moral heft, and it might be more compelling than the privacy-rights claim. In that case, the most parsimonious course of action would be to deny that there is a right to genetic privacy; the second-most would be to admit that there is a right, but it is inert. And the most parsimonious course is much less perplexing.

Notes

1 I shall have little directly to say about relational autonomy models here, since they tend to ride on the idea that information is confined.
2 Parker, M, & Lucassen, A, "Genetic Information: A Joint Account?" *British Medical Journal* 329[7458] (2004), p 166; cf Lucassen, A, & Parker, M, "Confidentiality and Sharing Genetic Information with Relatives", *The Lancet* 375[9725] (2010), p 1508.
3 Parker, M, & Lucassen, A, "Using a Genetic Test Result in the Care of Family Members: How Does the Duty of Confidentiality Apply?" *European Journal of Human Genetics* 26 (2018), *passim*.
4 Parker & Lucassen, *op cit* (2004), p 166.
5 Loi, M, "Direct to Consumer Genetic Testing and the Libertarian Right to Test", *Journal of Medical Ethics* 42[9] (2016), p 575.
6 *vide* Gilbar, R, & Foster, C, "Doctors' Liability to the Patient's Relatives in Genetic Medicine", *Medical Law Review* 24[1] (2015); Foster, C, & Gilbar, R, "Is There a New Duty to Warn Family Members in English Medical Law? ABC v St George's Healthcare NHS Trust and Others [2020] EWHC 455", *Medical Law Review* 29[2] (2021), *passim*.
7 Parker & Lucassen, *op cit* (2004), p 166.
8 Parker & Lucassen, *op cit* (2004), p 167; cf Lucassen, A *et al*, "Genetic Testing of Children: The Need for a Family Perspective", *American Journal of Bioethics* 14[3] (2014), *passim*.
9 Husted, J, "Autonomy and the Right Not to Know", in Chadwick, R *et al* (eds), *The Right to Know and the Right Not to Know* (Cambridge: Cambridge UP, 2014), pp 24–25 and *passim*.

10 Rhodes, R, "Confidentiality, Genetic Information, and the Physician-Patient Relationship", *American Journal of Bioethics* 1[3] (2001), p 27.

11 *ibid*, pp 27–28.

12 Liao, SM, "Is There a Duty to Share Genetic Information?" *Journal of Medical Ethics* 35[5] (2009), p 309.

13 Juth, N, "The Right Not to Know and the Duty to Tell: The Case of Relatives", *Journal of Law, Medicine & Ethics* 42[1] (2014), pp 47–48.

14 Parker, M, "Genetics and the Interpersonal Elaboration of Ethics", *Theoretical Medicine and Bioethics* 22[5] (2001), p 452.

15 Liukko, J, "Genetic Discrimination, Insurance, and Solidarity: An Analysis of the Argumentation for Fair Risk Classification", *New Genetics and Society* 29[4] (2010), p 458.

16 Genetic Information Nondiscrimination Act of 2008, sec 101 (emphasis mine).

17 A similar point is made by Jonathan Pugh in his "Genetic Information, Insurance and a Pluralistic Approach to Justice", *Journal of Medical Ethics* 47[4] (2021).

18 Americans with Disabilities Act 1990, sec. 12201.

19 Fiering, E, "Reassessing Insurers' Access to Genetic Information: Genetic Privacy, Ignorance, and Injustice", *Bioethics* 23[5] (2008), *passim*.

20 HM Government & Association of British Insurers, *Concordat and Moratorium on Genetics and Insurance* (London: Department of Health, 2005), § 19.

21 This statement had been published on the ABI's website at https://www.abi.org. uk/media/releases/2011/04/insurance_genetics_moratorium_extended_to_2017. aspx; by the time of writing, that link was dead, though the statement has been reported elsewhere: see, for example, https://www.insurancejournal.com/news/ international/2011/04/08/193782.htm.

22 HM Government & Association of British Insurers *Code on Genetic Testing and Insurance* Association of British Insurers, 2018; available via https://www.abi.org. uk/data-and-resources/tools-and-resources/genetics/code-on-genetic-testing-and- insurance/

23 *ibid*, p 14. The independent review process is initiated by the insurers, which may raise questions about just how independent it is; but it seems reasonable to suppose that were reasonable grounds given for thinking it to be other than independent, its recommendation would be set aside.

24 Chen, H, "Tay-Sachs Disease", in Chen, H (ed.), *Atlas of Genetic Diagnosis and Counseling* (2017), doi: 10.1007/978-1-4939-2401-1_225, p 2725.

25 Genetic Information Nondiscrimination Act of 2008. 42 USC 2000f, at 882.

26 Cancer Research UK, "Inherited Genes and Cancer Types" (2021), via https:// www.cancerresearchuk.org/about-cancer/causes-of-cancer/inherited-cancer-genes- and-increased-cancer-risk/inherited-genes-and-cancer-types

27 *vide* Leigh, S, "The Freedom to Underwrite", in Sorell, T (ed), *Health Care, Ethics and Insurance* (London: Routledge, 1998), esp pp 13–18; Collinson, P, "Rainbow Warrior in Stormy Waters", *The Guardian*, 12.i.2002, via https://www. theguardian.com/guardian_jobs_and_money/story/0,,631101,00.html; Massow, I, "The Downfall of the Man who Pioneered Affordable Insurance Cover for Homosexuals", *Daily Mail* 22.ix.2007, via https://www.dailymail.co.uk/news/ article-483299/The-downfall-man-pioneered-affordable-insurance-cover- homosexuals.html; Anon, "The Rise and Fall of Ivan Massow", *MoneyWeek*, 3.v.2007, via https://moneyweek.com/31642/the-rise-and-fall-of-ivan-massow; Cobb, N, "Queer(ed) Risks: Life Insurance, HIV/AIDS, and the 'Gay Question'", *Journal of Law and Society* 37[4] (2010), *passim*. That said, Leigh reported in 1998 (at p 18) that a gay HIV-negative man in a stable relationship could at that point still expect to pay an extra £3 p/a per £1000 assured, presumably just for being gay. In 2022, words like "gay" or "homosexual" do not

generate any useful results on the ABI website; "gay insurance" brings up over a thousand. Either way, results are too few or too many to be usefully specific, from which I infer that nobody thinks it relevant any more. (Sexuality's being a protected characteristic under the Human Rights Act will have contributed to this, but it is also reasonable to assume that an industry as powerful as insurance could have carved out a niche had it really seen a reason to do so; *modus tollens*, there was no reason.)

28 vide Association of British Insurers, ABI Guiding Principles for HIV and Life Insurance July 2016 (London: ABI, 2016), *passim*.

29 Birds, J, "The Current Law", in Tyldesley, P (ed), *Consumer Insurance Law: Disclosure, Representations and Basis of the Contract Clauses* (Haywards Heath: Bloomsbury Professional, 2013), p 6 (slightly modified).

30 Whether we *want* a free market in insurance, or at least to have to rely on such a market, is another matter: I'll have something more to say about that in a little while.

31 This is an appropriation and repurposing of a phrase coined by Charles Fried (1976) to describe the relationship between a lawyer and his client.

32 For a recent example of arguments along these lines, see Dempsey, J, "Corporations and Non-Agential Moral Responsibility", *Journal of Applied Philosophy* 30[4] (2013), and Dubbink, W, & Smith, J, "A Political Account of Corporate Moral Responsibility", *Ethical Theory and Moral Practice* 14[2] (2011), pp 223–246, each of which supplements an intriguing argument with a good list of the voluminous literature on this topic. See also Sepinwall, A, "Denying Corporate Rights and Punishing Corporate Wrongs", *Business Ethics Quarterly* 25[4] (2015); Sepinwall, A, "Corporate Moral Responsibility", *Philosophy Compass* 11[1] (2016), pp 3–13; and Sollars, G, "The Corporation: Genesis, Identity, Agency", in Heath, E *et al* (eds), *The Routledge Companion to Business Ethics* (London: Routledge, 2018).

33 As an aside, Ben Davies makes a related appeal to the interests of others as providing a duty to know about one's one genome, when ignorance (and, presumably, the inability to act in certain ways) would have a detrimental effect on others' interests: see "The Right Not to Know and the Obligation to Know", *Journal of Medical Ethics* 46[5] (2020). Clearly, this is a repudiation of Laurevian "push" privacy.

34 Fricker, M, *Epistemic Injustice: Power and the Ethics of Knowing* (Oxford: Oxford UP, 2007), p 4.

35 *ibid*, p 7.

36 *ibid*, p 20.

37 *ibid*, p 2.

38 Rawls, J, *Political Liberalism* (New York: Columbia UP, 2005), p 267.

39 McGee, A, *The Modern Law of Insurance* (London: LexisNexis Butterworths, 2011), p 74.

40 Hoy, M, & Witt, J, "Welfare Effects of Banning Genetic Information in the Life Insurance Market: The Case of BRCA1/2 Genes", *The Journal of Risk and Insurance* 74[3] (2007), p 525 (emphasis mine).

41 *ibid*, p 536.

42 Evans, J *et al*, "Genetic Exceptionalism: Too Much of a Good Thing?" *Genetics in Medicine* 10[7] (2008), p 500.

43 A similar point is made by Thomas Murray in his "Genetics and the Moral Mission of Health Insurance", *The Hastings Center Report* 22[6] (1992), p 17.

44 Eli Feiring concludes that "[i]f or when predictive medical tests, such as genetic tests, are developed with significant actuarial value [there is] a good case for abandoning the health insurance market in favour of a universal health care system based on solidarity, where the level of cover is associated with the level of

medical need": see "Reassessing Insurers' Access to Genetic Information: Genetic Privacy, Ignorance, and Injustice", *Bioethics* 23[5] (2009), p 309.

45 See Brassington, I, "On Rights of Inheritance and Bequest", *Journal of Ethics* 23[2] (2019), *passim* for more on this.

46 de Groot, N *et al*, "Accessing Medical Biobanks to Solve Crimes: Ethical Considerations", *Journal of Medical Ethics* 47[12] (2021), *passim*.

47 https://www.gedmatch.com/about-us.

48 Zabel, J, "The Killer Inside Us: Law, Ethics, and the Forensic Use of Family Genetics", *Berkeley Journal of Criminal Law* 24[2] (2019), pp 50–51.

49 See, for example, Feeney, M, "'Genetic Informants' and the Hunt for the Golden State Killer" (Cato Institute, 2018) via https://www.cato.org/blog/genetic-informants-hunt-golden-state-killer; Kolata, G, & Murphy, H, "The Golden State Killer Is Tracked through a Thicket of DNA, and Experts Shudder", *New York Times*, 27.iv.2018, via https://www.nytimes.com/2018/04/27/health/dna-privacy-golden-state-killer-genealogy.html; Scutti, S, "What the Golden State Killer Case Means for Your Genetic Privacy", CNN 26.iv.2018, via https://edition.cnn.com/2018/04/27/health/golden-state-killer-genetic-privacy/index.html

50 Guerrini, CJ *et al* "Should Police Have Access to Genetic Genealogy Databases? Capturing the Golden State Killer and Other Criminals Using a Controversial New Forensic Technique", *PLoS Biology* 16[10] (2018), *passim*; Wickenheiser, R, "Forensic Genealogy, Bioethics and the Golden State Killer Case", *Forensic Science International: Synergy* 1 (2019), pp 144–125, *passim*.

51 Greytak, E *et al*, "Privacy and Genetic Genealogy Data", *Science* 361[6405] (2018), p 857.

52 Guerrini *et al*, *op cit*, p 2.

53 For arguments in favour of such a databank, see Kaye, D, "Two Fallacies about DNA Data Banks for Law Enforcement", *Brooklyn Law Review* 67[1] (2001); Kaye, D, & Smith, M, "DNA Identification Databases: Legality, Legitimacy, and the Case for Population-Wide Coverage", *Wisconsin Law Review* 2003[3] (2003); Dedrickson, K, "Universal DNA Databases: A Way to *Improve* Privacy?" *Journal of Law and the Biosciences* 4[3] (2018); and Hazel, J *et al*, "Is It Time for a Universal Genetic Forensic Database?" *Science* 362[6417] (2018); for a highly readable rebuttal of this genus of argument, see Krimsky, S, & Simoncelli, T, *Genetic Justice: DNA Databanks, Criminal Investigations, and Civil Liberties* (New York: Columbia UP, 2012), esp. §8.

54 Postan, E, *Embodied Narratives: Protecting Identity Interests through Ethical Governance of Bioinformation* (Cambridge: Cambridge UP, 2022), p 182.

Part III

Rebuilding Genetic Privacy Rights

7 Reinventing Privacy

i. Sense and Reference and Rights

Genetic privacy, and any right to it, is slippery. The Gerry and Terry problem is slightly contrived, but it does allow light to be thrown onto some of genetic privacy's problems; in so doing, it forces us to admit that there may be good reasons either to make exceptions to intuitive norms, which seems *ad hoc*, or to wonder whether informational privilege really is all that privileged. If we want to hold on to the idea of genetic privacy tightly, we ought to be careful that it does not become something other than privacy under the pressure. Some may want to insist that Gerry and Terry's situation is exceptional because they are identical twins. But I have also suggested that this is not so: their being monozygotic throws problems into relief, but those problems are much more general. Given that, the main theories of privacy do not seem to apply all that well to genetic information, and that there may be good moral reasons to discount some genetic privacy rights claims in favour of accessibility.

Further, honesty forces us to admit that third parties such as insurers do have interests in being able to access genetic information, either on their own behalf or on behalf of other stakeholders and policyholders. Even if we are still satisfied that private insurers ought not to have access to genetic information, or that they should have access only on very limited terms, the proposition that they should have it at all needs to be taken seriously, and argued against. By implication, something similar would apply in respect of other agents, be they individuals or institutions, who may have an interest in information about another's genome. This point obviously speaks to real-life situations such as the ABC case or the use of genetic information in finding and prosecuting the perpetrators of crimes. There may be times when third parties have an entitlement to more information about our genomes than we would initially have thought, and when they have an entitlement to more than we would like, based in their having a particular interest in that information. Once we accept that it is the measuring and comparing of interests that is crucial in determining the enforceability of a putative right to privacy, we find that we do

DOI: 10.4324/9781003312512-11

not need to appeal to rights anyway, and the difficulties of defining them appropriately and of stating them meaningfully evaporate.

Lest it appear that I am moving much too quickly with this, and helping myself to far too much, it's worth spending a few paragraphs considering not a right to privacy, but what I take to be going on when we talk about rights *at all*, and so filling out some of the claims I made in the last chapter. The common-or-garden conception of a right is that it is a *datum* of moral debate, generating moral reasons for action or inaction: a question like "Why should I do or refrain from this?" can be met with an answer along the lines of "Because I have a right that you do or refrain from it", and that answer will be adequate to motivate the behaviour that the right-holder desires. For Alice to have a right to some φ means either – negatively – that Bob has a reason (whether or not he knows it at the time) not to prevent Alice's φ-ing or accessing φ, or – positively – that Bob has a reason (whether or not he knows it at the time) to assist Alice's φ-ing or accessing φ. Put another way, on this kind of account, a right is a kind of moral reason.[1] What supposedly distinguishes a right from other kinds of moral reason is that a right has a peremptory force; and it has that peremptory force just because it is a right. The difficulties lie in distinguishing between reasons that are rights-related and reasons that are not: when claims conflict, the proponent of each will naturally think that his position has peremptory force because it stems from some right that he has. Gerry and Terry will both want to claim that they have a right to control information about them, and that that right will mean that the other ought to give ground.

This is a problem articulated by John Mackie. He defines a right as "the conjunction of a freedom and a claim-right", by which he means that

> if someone, A, has the moral right to do X, not only is he entitled to do X if he chooses – he is not morally required not to do X – but he is also protected in his doing of X – others are morally required not to interfere or prevent him.[2]

However, he also notes that "[t]he rights we have assigned to all persons will in practice come into conflict with one another", and that "[o]ne person's choice of how to live will constantly be interfering with the choices of others".[3] And this fact leads him to suppose that "the rights we have called fundamental can be no more than *prima facie* rights: the rights that in the end people have, their final rights, must result from compromises between their initially conflicting rights".[4]

Mackie concedes that there would be vital interests that would be sacrosanct, providing fixed points around which the network of rights would be woven. However, he also suggests that the "shape" of the network would depend on the details of the negotiators:

> [W]e might think in terms of a model in which each person is represented by a point-center of force, and the forces (representing

prima facie rights) obey an inverse square law, so that a right decreases in weight with the remoteness of the matter on which it bears from the person whose right it is. There will be some matters so close to each person that, with respect to them, his rights will nearly always outweigh any aggregate of other rights, though admittedly it will sometimes happen that issues arise in which the equally vital interests of two or more people clash.[5]

It is important to note in all this that the *prima facie* rights of which Mackie speaks are in a sense "provisional" – they are, as it were, opening bids that draw on interests that we may have or wish to pursue, some of which will be vital, and others not. But this does raise at least a few questions.

First, if they are only *prima facie*, and if at least some of these interests will be trumped by others, why refer to them as rights at all? Why not just talk about them as interests, or claimed rights, or candidate rights, or something like that? When Mackie raises the possibility that two persons' equally vital interests may clash, this does seem to invite us to invent a right rather than discover it: talking in terms of *ab initio* rights would be less welcoming to this, since by implication we could not help but to violate one or both agents' rights, which suggests a wrong. Sticking to the language of interests tracks more closely what we are constrained to think morality requires in such situations. Second, where is the threshold between rights and other reasons? To take Mackie's inverse-square analogy, at what (presumably non-arbitrary) "distance" does a consideration exert sufficient force that it becomes proper to think of it as a right? Third, what is the status of *prima facie* rights that lose out to other *prima facie* rights? Do they still have any persuasive force, such that they could perhaps moderate how those surviving rights are exercised? If they do, what is the precise difference between having a right – *prima facie* or otherwise – and being able to present others with concomitant reasons to act in a particular way, and being able to present others with more common-or-garden reasons to act in a particular way under any other circumstance?

Others hold that rights that act as "trumps" in moral, political, and legal debate. Under a "rights as trumps" account, to assert a right is not just to articulate a moral reason that others should take seriously: if someone has a right to φ, then it is wrong for others to prevent that φ, and will always be wrong, irrespective of the circumstance.[6] (This is a parallel to the kind of thing that Nozick has in mind when he talks about rights as "side constraints"[7]: they are barriers that keep moral and political arguments on the track, rather as the walls of a bobsleigh track stop the vehicle shooting off to where it shouldn't go.) Conversely, if a putative right is itself trumped and so loses its normative force in the face of other social or moral goals, it is reasonable to say that *modus tollens* it is not a right after all. Dworkin articulates a way for this idea to work:

> We might, for simplicity, stipulate not to call any political aim a right unless it has a certain threshold weight against collective goals in

general; unless, for example, it cannot be defeated by appeal to any of the ordinary routine goals of political administration, but only by a goal of special urgency. Suppose, for example, some man says he recognizes the right of free speech, but adds that free speech must yield whenever its exercise would inconvenience the public. He means, I take it, that he recognizes the pervasive goal of collective welfare, and only such distribution of liberty of speech as that collective goal recommends in particular circumstances. His political position is exhausted by the collective goal; the putative right adds nothing and there is no point to recognizing it as a right at all.[8]

There is a difference between something's *being* a right and its *being recognised as* a right, admittedly; but what really matters here is that if a putative right has to fight for precedence over other moral principles, then it does not really have the special status that the word "right" normally implies. We lose nothing by treating it as a moral reason or a moral principle among others. And this may be desirable, because it keeps debates simple and – for want of a better word – honest. Calling something a right from the off is the rhetorical equivalent of keeping one's thumb on the scales.

Yet Mackie's point still nags. There may be certain things that really are indisputably rights, and in respect of which there could never be a clash of competing interests. I am inclined to think, for example, that our recognising another person *as* a person means recognising them as a moral equal; and to this extent, they occupy a certain moral position that means that while I may discount some of their interests in respect of my own, I cannot discount *them*. As such, a person has a right to equality of esteem inasmuch as that is a part of recognising him as a moral agent at all. This is a fairly orthodox line of thought; but much beyond that the possibility of a clash of putative rights is likely to become nontrivial fairly quickly – and certainly in respect of problems of who has access to what genetic information and on what terms. Gerry and Terry can perfectly easily recognise that the other has a dignity beyond price, and that dignity beyond price might well in some way be the foundation of a claim to informational privilege; but that doesn't help resolve disputes all that much, since it applies to both. Both might claim a right to control the information; as such, it is not clear what is gained by using the language of "rights", except as a rhetorical device. The alternative is to say that each has a right, but that they are equal and opposite, and that they cancel each other out. Again, though, we would be none the wiser about what to do. *Mutatis mutandis*, the same kind of impasse will be arrived at in the Kerry and Perry scenario, or any situation in which agents might claim either competing rights, or competing applications of the same right.

These problems (and the problems of finding a robust theoretical account of privacy rights that stretches to genetics) can be avoided if we abandon the idea that rights to genetic privacy are axiomatic and have a place at the beginning of moral discussion. I shall assume that Mackie's picture reflects something more accurate, which is that a right such as a right to genetic privacy is whatever we are left with when the moral argument is done. By assessing the principles in play in respect of a given decision, we can decide what rights obtain. Kerry has a right to genetic privacy – a right to prevent Perry accessing certain genetic information – if, all things considered, Perry's interests in accessing her information pale in comparison to Kerry's interest in not sharing it. Rather as Mackie's "inverse square" model of *prima facie* rights can only be applied meaningfully when we are considering the relationship between two point-centres of force and the way they interact with each other, the question of who has what rights can only ever be approached case-by-case and in the light of interactions with others. As such, a person might be held to have a privacy right in respect of some people at some times, but not in respect of all people at all times; a right to privacy – certainly a right to genetic privacy – is on this account a product of the relationships between agents and their claims on each other. (Writing in a different but obviously pertinent context, Kevin Mills makes a point that surely translates to this position:

(It has long been recognized in the literature on the right to privacy that people do not have a right to absolute privacy; they have a right to reasonable privacy, and what counts as reasonable privacy is determined by balancing people's privacy interests against those various interests of others with which they conflict. The scope and limits of the access right, assuming it is a genuine right at all, depend on the independent justifications that can be offered for and against various data practices.[9])

A rough parallel here may be drawn with the ways in which we may think about money. On an everyday level, we tend to think about money as being a prerequisite of economic interactions, and as something that we may choose to exchange for goods and services. However, a more accurate view of money is that it is nothing but the product of an intricate web of credit and debt; it is the outcome of economic interaction, rather than its basis.[10] My claim about rights to genetic privacy works in a similar way[11]: these rights are ways to talk about and keep track of a web of obligations and standards of decency owed by agents to each other, rather than determinants of obligation and decency.

This does not commit us to eliminativism about rights, or to abandoning the language of rights. There are lots of concepts that have a useful role to play in everyday conversation, even if they turn out to refer to other things, or even if they turn out not to have any extension at all: sense is not reference. We can talk about money in the familiar ways even if we know that it is the product, rather than a prerequisite, of economic interactions; and replacing the word "money" with something more supposedly accurate will hinder rather than advance talking about those interactions. In just the same way, a term like "privacy rights" *does* have a place in everyday speech about genetic information. It plays a role in the language.

All of which raises a question: what are the principles that determine the proper use of genetic information? What are the terms of the debate?

ii. Principlism and Respect for Autonomy

For better or worse, Beauchamp and Childress's "four principles" – beneficence, non-maleficence, respect for autonomy, and justice – have become prevalent in bioethical discussion, and so when we're asking what the principles that guide decisionmaking about genetic information should be, it makes sense to start with them – partly because they're there, central to the standard model with which a good many practitioners will be familiar, and partly because principlism is really only a way to articulate fairly basic ideas anyway.

"Principlism" ought not to be understood as a normative theory, and I shall not treat it as such now. What became known in some circles as the "Georgetown Mantra" should be understood as an attempt to capture the distilled essence of a putative "common morality" encompassing the kinds of thing that everyone would expect to see thrown up by any recognisable moral theory.[12] As such, principlism provides a fairly thin account of morality. In one sense, this is its virtue; but it means that there is still work to do in thickening it for practical application. For example, nobody would deny that "justice" names a good; but what counts as justice will be disputable. Similarly, it is open also to ask what "respect for autonomy" entails: whether it's supposed to mean that autonomy is more important than the other principles, or whether it means simply that it's something we should keep in mind. When Raanan Gillon insists that respect for autonomy is "first among equals" of the principles,[13] we might still wonder whether he is correct (Beauchamp and Childress would not endorse the claim[14]), and what the standard is by which we should assess this sort of claim in the first place.

Resisting the temptation to treat this (or any) set of principles as a complete normative theory allows us to look at it in its best light, as offering a way to understand the nature of our dilemmas. They help articulate moral reasons, rather than generating them; and there is accordingly no particular reason why a thorough understanding of the principles in play in a given situation would, in itself, bring us much closer to understanding what we ought to do, except inasmuch as that we would perhaps have a clearer idea of the competing candidates. As such, I will not in this chapter be attempting to offer any account of how to solve any particular dilemma about the control of genetic information; still, I hope to be able to cast light on what makes it a dilemma at all. Circumstance, and our own dispositions, will suggest which principle – and which interpretation of which principle – is the more important; but even that is subject to modification through processes of public reasoning (about which I shall have a little more to say at the end of this chapter).

I have dealt with autonomy (and respect for it) implicitly at some length up to this point. Intuitions about informational privilege are inseparable from the liberal idea that we should be able to have the fullest possible control over our lives, and to exclude others from our lives and ourselves from theirs if we wish. That Gerry might have an entitlement to access information about himself in order that he can put that information to use in his own life is a *sequela* of that idea; so is any sympathy that we have for Terry. I take it as obvious that we have a reason to consider what people would prefer to happen when making decisions about whether to share genetic information, or about who should have access to it and under what circumstances. Nevertheless, it would be naïve to think that this exhausts the debate. And even if one happens to think that respect for autonomy is *generally* the most important moral principle, one would not be committed to the idea that it *always* is; even if one thinks that it is the most important single principle in any particular situation, one would not be committed to the idea that it cannot occasionally be overshadowed by a combination of other principles; even if one thinks that it is always the most important principle in any dilemma, one could still accept that it might play out in several incompatible ways. All in all, appeals to respect for autonomy are not all that normatively significant. Were we *not* to respect autonomy, many of the problems about access to information would never arise – we could be naïve utilitarians, for example. The problem is that respect for autonomy is at the root of many of the problems that we face: thinking that we can solve them by respecting autonomy a bit more is unhelpful at best.

iii. Non-Maleficence and Beneficence

Who would argue for maleficence? The absurdity of taking anything other than an anti-maleficence position gives gravitational pull to the idea that it is the least useful of the Georgetown Four. Upon examination, there is a little more to the principle; yet while a more charitable reading of it shows that it is not entirely trivial, it is still a little short on utility when it comes to addressing practical questions about who should have control over what genetic information and on what terms.

The principle of non-maleficence articulates, fundamentally, a general norm against causing harm; but it could also be taken as a more general principle of harm-aversion. The difficulty is that inflicting harm on others may sometimes be an unavoidable part of healthcare, and not an especial cause for regret. It is not difficult to give examples of situations in which it may be permissible to inflict harm for the sake of realising some greater good: a vaccine may cause a passing fever, but we would not want to say that there was anything impermissible about the vaccination; giving blood is time-consuming, a little uncomfortable, and might make us faint, yet it is not wild to think that these are setbacks that one ought to tolerate, as undesirable-but-inescapable aspects of things that one ought to endorse; participants in research trials may be at risk of injury, but this may not be too worrisome all things considered. Merely putting someone at risk, irrespective of whether any actual injury manifests, could well also count as a harm, since it is better not to be at risk. So might a setback in their interests.

Beauchamp and Childress observe that "no rule in ethics favors avoiding harm over providing benefit in every circumstance",[15] and on any reasonable account of action, this must be true. Sometimes benefits outweigh harms, and a naïve adherence to a principle of non-maleficence would generate counterintuitive outcomes. When the problem is a conflict between agents over control of information in which one must suffer a setback to his interests – as it would be when one person wants access to genetic information that the other would prefer withheld – it is inescapable. Terry or Kerry might be harmed by having had their genetic information accessed, and Gerry and Perry (or Perry's clients) may be harmed by privacy being treated as trumps.

Perhaps the idea is that one should not cause harm unless doing so would avoid a grave setback – that there are some harms that are so great as to mean that there would be no overarching good that could count against them, and some courses of action that nobody could endorse outside of the seminar-room. Quite possibly, there could be times when there would be enormous harm done by sharing information that could not be counterbalanced by any good outcome. But there could also be times when the reverse is true.

How are we to draw the moral line, though? One possible answer to that question would be to say that the impermissible causation of harm involves a violation of rights. This would certainly explain how it is that killing one person to save two others would attract moral disapprobation, and how a vaccination that we expect will give the recipient a fever probably would not. But this is not a move that is available to me when it comes to deciding how to work out the proper course of action in respect of genetic information, because my hypothesis is that rights are not *data* in moral debate. If rights – or, at the very least, rights to genetic privacy – are to be ascribed as an outcome of moral debate, they cannot be things that we consider in the course of deriving that outcome. Besides, if we are inclined to think that rights *are* among the *data* of moral debate and that they are the thing that distinguishes the permissible from the impermissible, then it becomes that much less clear why we should worry all that much about non-maleficence *qua* non-maleficence anyway: it is a person's rights that will do the moral heavy lifting.

Another possible move would be to capitalise on the observation that there is a difference between acting in a way such as to cause harm, and acting in a way such as to cause harm intentionally, and to distinguish on that basis between maleficence and malevolence. A principle of non-malevolence would articulate an injunction against wilfully harmful behaviour. It would suggest that we should worry not so much about harm being caused by the sharing or withholding of genetic information – since there may be better or worse reasons for that – as about its being shared or withheld *malevolently*. Even if one were incompetently malevolent, and somehow ended up making the world better, one would still be blameable.

But while malevolent action will always be morally troubling, drawing this distinction will not be of much help. One of the most obvious reasons for this is that while such a move captures the intuition that the intention to harm is morally wrong, a principle of non-malevolence really is so obvious as not to be worth stating. For this reason, it would neither explain the origin of, nor help us formulate a response to, genuine moral dilemmas: a psychologically plausible person who has to decide in good faith whether or not to hand over a certain piece of genetic information to the police will never be wondering whether or not to do the malevolent or the non-malevolent thing. They may misidentify the right thing; but trying to decide whether or not to do something that they recognise as malevolent or malicious is the province of the moustache-twiddling cartoon villain. And the possibility of failure to identify the right thing helps locate another objection, which is that sometimes well-meaning actions can be blameable if they are carried out naively or if they contravene moral claims that we ought to take seriously. For example, a student who provides answers to a colleague to help him pass an exam may have been well-meaning, but we would still be inclined to say that he has acted wrongfully. If we decide that, all things considered, Perry ought not to have been given access to Kerry's genetic information, there is still no reason to suppose that anyone acted malevolently.

And so the principle of non-maleficence captures a morally relevant consideration when deciding how to handle genetic information, but not as something that is likely to be definitive one way or the other. Avoiding harm, widely defined, will be impossible in situations in which claims conflict and neither claimant can be satisfied without causing some setback to the other. However, the important consideration will not be whether or not harm is caused, but whether it is gratuitous or unnecessarily grave. Some account would have to be forthcoming of what is necessary, what is unnecessary, and what is gratuitous; and though distinguishing the gratuitous from the non-gratuitous is likely to be straightforward and general enough, what is necessary and what is not is likely to change on a case-by-case basis. This should not worry us. There are likely to be general patterns drawn from experience and a general familiarity with the way such epithets are applied in everyday language that will guide us when it comes to deciding whether they should be applied in a given case. Beyond that, it would be surprising if there were a neat template that we could apply.

These considerations can be drawn on and re-used to facilitate a fairly quick analysis of the principle of beneficence, which at its most basic suggests a moral obligation to improve the world, but could also mean that we are under a general obligation to ensure that the world is as good a place as possible. Beauchamp and Childress themselves touch on a distinction between beneficence and benevolence, albeit without capitalising on it, when they suggest that benevolence "refers to the character trait of being disposed to act for the benefit of others", whereas beneficence relates to "mercy, kindness, friendship, charity, and the like".[16] But the difficulty with all this is that it is possible to wrong or harm a person, or to make the world as a whole worse in some way, with the best of intentions; and when it comes to information, it is very easy to see how an agent might decide that the harm generated by sharing is more than mitigated by the benefit that accrues to, or the harm that would be avoided by, some other identifiable person. Alternatively, we could envisage situations in which an agent might think nothing of sharing information for the best possible reasons without it occurring that there may be interests set back. For example, what would the beneficent or benevolent thing have been in a case like *Tarasoff*? I ask this wholly rhetorically: the point is that either sharing or not sharing the information could be argued to be the more beneficent or benevolent option. Much the same could be said in respect of the situation facing the medical staff who had been looking after XX in ABC, or of the Gerry and Terry case: it is not clear what beneficence would dictate. In the Kerry and Perry case, it is tempting to think that Kerry's position is the one more easily squared with the demands of beneficence – but there is a good to be derived from sharing information, and all things considered, it may be greater than the good of privacy. At the very least, that is an arguable position to adopt. Finally, we might consider cases in which an agent decides to contribute to some medical research programme that will make use of information about his genome; in choosing to participate, he will have – in effect – opened up the genome of his relatives, or perhaps a wider group such as a tribe, to scrutiny, quite possibly without the permission of these indirect referents: what should we say about beneficence and benevolence here?

It is a further question as to whether there really is a moral obligation to generate the best possible outcome anyway. That there is an obligation not to make the world worse, or at least not to be indifferent to its becoming worse, is fairly easy to argue. That there is a *reason* to make it better is also fairly easy to argue. However, not all reasons are obligations; and there could be situations in which the course of action that does not make the world better would be the morally right one. If we think that privacy is sufficiently important, we might think that we ought to pass on the opportunity to improve the world materially if that improvement is privacy-violating. Or consider ABC again, and suppose that the medical staff (to whom, for the sake of this part of the argument, we can ascribe perfect knowledge and predictive abilities) were satisfied that the world's stock of welfare would have been maximised by revealing information about ABC's father's genetic profile to her. Even so, it is perfectly plausible to say that though the optimificity of sharing is *a reason* to share, it is less important morally speaking than, say, honouring an explicit commitment not to; and I shall have more to say about such commitments in a moment, when I consider a principle of fidelity. Not everyone will agree with this assessment; but it is still arguable. I would contend that someone who tries to discount the value of the promise either simply because it is not optimific, or on the basis that the value of promise-keeping is that it is in the end optimific itself, is not thinking about morality and conduct in a particularly rich or, when it comes to it, plausible way. But even putting that contention to one side, the point would stand that there is a range of courses of action that might be held to satisfy a principle of beneficence; and plenty of courses of action where we might argue about whether that principle is satisfied.

iv. Justice

Questions about justice in bioethics are often about who gets how much of a limited resource, and when, and who foots the bill. If there is a justice aspect to problems of genetic information, this picture is less straightforward, one important reason for which is that information is not a limited resource. Quite the opposite: the more information is shared, the more of it there is. If Fred and George are candidates for a heart transplant and there is only one heart, then what Fred gets George doesn't. But giving information to Perry does not deprive Kerry of any information that she might otherwise have had.

At the core of the problem is a question not about who has access to a limited resource and what opportunity is lost by the other, but about who has *control* over the resource. Whatever its shortcomings in respect of genetics, the CoPI account of privacy rights is on the right track here. If the information is given to Perry, then Kerry will have lost control of it; if Kerry does not want to surrender control of the information, she will be disposed not to share it. It is not that there is one discrete "lump" of control that is held by one or the other – Kerry could choose to disclose the information to Perry on condition that Perry not disseminate it further, or on the basis that she only use it for certain purposes – and so the matter is not wholly binary. But the more control over the information is held by one of the two, the less is held by the other; and much the same would apply in most other cases in which there is a problem about the distribution of genetic information. (The Gerry and Terry problem seems to be an instance in which the options are much more binary: either Terry has control of the information, or Gerry does, and that's that. But insofar as that there will be questions about what any one person may do with unconfined information from which others may be identified, even here things are not simple: we may want to say that an agent may do some things, but not others, and that one would only be able to claim complete control and liberty in respect of information if, *per impossibile*, one had no blood relatives at all.)

And so here is one way in which we can talk about the justice or injustice of a decision about who gets access to genetic information or who gets to use it or decide on its use: there is a distribution of control that has to be managed. When it comes to deciding on the just distribution, a tolerably Rawlsian account looks promising: what we would call a just distribution of control – which is a just distribution of power – is that which rational self-interested observers would accept as binding them were they deprived of knowledge about their relationship to that information. An important reason for this is that Rawls is clear that political rights are *assigned* rather than discovered, and arise from a process of discussion in the "original position" – and so his position is similar to the one that I shall have sketched out by the end of this chapter.[17]

The framework of the Rawlsian account of justice – in which basic liberties are protected so that everyone has as much basic liberty as possible compatibly with everyone else having the same entitlement, and social and economic inequalities are arranged to provide the greatest possible benefit to the least advantaged all under conditions of fair equality of opportunity[18] – is augmented by an appeal to important "primary goods", the recognition of which Rawls holds to be necessary for citizens to be recognised as free and equal agents able to pursue life of their own.[19] These five goods are basic rights and liberties; freedom of movement and choice in occupation; income and wealth; the social bases of self-respect; and what he dubs the "powers and prerogatives of offices and positions of responsibility in political and economic institutions" – essentially, the ability to access politically important roles.[20] But Rawls does not claim that this list is complete, and van den Hoven and Rooksby suggest that access to information is a good that is necessary to a person carrying out a complete plan of life, adding a sixth good to Rawls's five.[21] This gives us a way to think about what justice would look like in respect of genetic information: decisions about who should have access to what information, and on what terms, ought to be decided on the basis of the impact that a given distribution would have on the freedom and equality of individuals.

But how ought we to understand "freedom and equality"? And, in the event that they pull apart – which they might, given that liberty may disrupt strict equality, and Rawls' own liberal state will tolerate inequality – which has priority? It is likely that the second of these questions dissolves once we begin to answer the first. Granted that "equality" requires treatment as an equal rather than naïve equal treatment, this means that justice requires equal consideration of the interests and welfare of all; in turn, that would set limits on the degree to which one may infringe on another's freedom (on the assumption that my recognising you as a moral equal implies that I have a moral reason to assume the same basic freedoms). Clearly, this point speaks to claims about the social basis of self-respect: a distribution of information or a rubric for distributing information will be incompatible with the demands of justice to the extent that it represents an erosion of the social – that is, interpersonal – basis of self-respect.

None of this will tell us directly how we ought to settle problems about who ought to have access to genetic information and when; but it does offer us a starting point. While the information available to someone like Gerry may make a difference to the *kind* of decision he makes and the range of options from which he can choose to make it, it does not follow that it makes a difference to whether or not he has autonomy or self-determination at all. On the other hand, it seems reasonable to suppose that Gerry might still be wronged by not having access to information that relates to his own life: and were Terry to seek to prevent his brother's accessing genetic information in order to influence his decisionmaking, that would be an instance of Terry's subordinating Gerry's status as an equal to his own. Terry's preference to maintain privacy would not count for nothing; but seen from the perspective of assessing justice, it would not be the whole story. Similarly, in respect of the Kerry and Perry problem, the question would be one of assessing what the best distribution of control over information would be, granted the competing interests in play – and seen from a Rawlsian perspective, the just distribution would have to take account of the fact that the holders of the competing interests are, *qua* agents, free and equal. (As we saw, this may involve other commitments: if Perry is considered to be simply a proxy for the firm, then this may lead us to think that one distribution of control is more just; if we think that she is speaking not for the shareholders but for the other policyholders, we may lean towards another.)

In *ABC*, the bare fact that XX preferred not to share information may not have wronged ABC; she could still have had a genetic test, or made reproductive decisions based on what she knew or suspected. But to the extent that XX wished information to be withheld from his daughter *in order to influence her reproductive decisions*, he did wrong her; this wrong counts as an instance of injustice, because it represents an attempt by XX to claim an unjust power over ABC – unjust because it would move the distribution of control away from what would be recognised as just by a community that recognises the freedom and moral equality of all.

The difficulty with a Rawlsian account is its generality. It is central to the account that justice is a function of fairness, and fairness can be determined by deliberators on the matter placing themselves behind a veil of ignorance, such that a fair distribution is that which would satisfy the maximinning principles of those deliberators. This is fair enough as a principle, and it may give us a reasonable way to think about the structures of a given society; but when it comes to real-life decisionmaking, it is plainly not much use. We cannot separate ourselves from our situation; even a notionally disinterested judge in a courtroom can only go through the motions of trying to work out what negotiators behind a veil of ignorance would decide ought to be the case – and he should not have to do this.

But we can strip things back further, and say that it is possible to arrive at judgements about what is just and what is fair based on nothing more than the analysis of language. On this account, what counts as a just distribution of access to information, or power in respect of information, depends less on trying to work out what rational self-interested people behind a veil of ignorance would choose, than on working out the distribution we would agree most readily is apt to be described as such. This is not empty or wishy-washy "justice is whatever you think it is" subjectivism: rather, the opposite. There is within natural languages a set of rules that determine whether a word is properly used; and in an important sense, there is nothing to knowing what a word means except knowing how to deploy it in language. We know whether a dancer's movement is graceful by calling on situations in which the word "graceful" has been used in the past, working out the pattern of the word's correct deployment hitherto, and applying it in line with that pattern. Whether our use of the word fits with this pattern determines whether it is correctly applied; our claims about grace will be deemed more or less accurate depending on how well we are deemed to have followed the pattern and whether our claims meet with disagreement, puzzlement, or outright bafflement. Accordingly, we can talk about a graceful dancer; and if she stumbles, we would withhold the epithet. If we describe the stumble as "graceful", others would be entitled to tell us that we had made a mistake – either we have missed some detail of what had just happened, or we are misusing the word. Similarly, we may be inclined to say that someone who talks about a graceful summer breeze is talking poetically or unclearly (which may amount to the same thing), that someone who talks about a graceful housebrick is mistaken about the English language, and that someone who talks about a graceful tumour is mad. Crucially, the work in determining whether a dancer (or a spring day, or a tumour) is or even can be graceful has already been done for us: it is built into the conceptual apparatus that we inherit as part of our ability to spot characteristics in the world and to fit them into a linguistic pattern. In other words, it is built into our being a competent user of whichever language we are speaking. By parity of reasoning, we can hope to say whether a proposed allocation of information or access or power over information is just by considering whether, based on the pattern of its use hitherto, we would describe it as such. If the word is apt, then the distribution is just; if it is not, it is not. What else do we need? On this sort of account, judgements are corrigible by analogy with other situations, be they real-world, literary, or wholly hypothetical. It is the work of pure analytic philosophy.

(Rawls' own framework is amenable to this kind of analysis. What is justice? Fairness. What is fairness? That which rational and self-interested deliberators behind a veil of ignorance would accept. And what makes this a plausible theory of fairness, and hence of justice? Simply that it fits the way those words are used in common English. His account of justice as fairness depends for its coherence on his presentation of the words "justice" and "fairness" in a certain way. If we think that Rawls is wrong, we demonstrate that by showing that, after all, a word like "fairness" is better applied in some other way.)

Still, whatever account we favour of how to judge justice, the important point is that we can talk about more or less just ways of dealing with genetic information; the key thing is that the question is less about who gets the information than it is about who gets *control* of the information – it is control, not information itself, that is finite. It is likely that justice will prove to be the highest-order principle, by which I mean that working out the just allocation of control of information will draw on conclusions we would already have drawn in respect of other moral principles. And in all this, not least because control speaks to power, and the power that one person may have over another, it is desirable to keep in mind that parties to a dispute about genetic information may not be meeting as equals. One person may be epistemically privileged over the other: for example, it might be that Kerry is wholly unaware of the importance of a particular gene when Perry asks her about it, and this may mean that she is not participating in discussions about access as an equal, and so may accept as fair something that a third party would not. Just as worries about the just allocation of tangible goods ought to keep in mind that that one party in any allocation dispute may well come to the table with more power to make his case than the other, and whatever the decision made will impact on the relative power relations of those parties, the same applies here. Power is not a bad thing – but it is both an input and an output of discussions about the just allocation of any good, tangible or intangible.

v. Power and the Limits of Justice

One further sense in which we might think about justice and power has to do with the distribution of power between those who have the ability to decide who has access to what information, and those in respect of whom the decision is made. Consider the archetypal information-sharing dilemma, such as in a case like *Tarasoff*, in which the patient obviously has the freedom to share information if he chooses. The problems arise if the patient would rather keep the information unshared, and the therapist is unsure about what to do. That it lies with the therapist to decide whether to share gives him a certain inescapable power over the patient, though: the patient is like a supplicant, whose request (implicit or explicit) that the information be kept within the confines of the therapeutic relationship is within the therapist's gift to grant or refuse. The same applies in respect of genetic information that is disclosed in the context of a consultation. Emma, the geneticist in the Gerry and Terry case, has the power to decide whose claim on the information is the stronger. Similarly, a woman who has been discovered to carry the BRCA-1 gene, or a father with Huntington's, may each say that they do not want anyone else to know about it; but irrespective of how good their reasons are, it is ultimately up to the medical staff dealing with her to decide what to do. There is, as a result, always a power difference between the practitioner and the client or patient.

This point takes us a little outside of the question of who should have access to genetic information and on what terms, but it is clearly related, since that question is one that the practitioner will have to face. Her relative power in this situation does not depend on any of the considerations I have spelled out in the last few paragraphs – it is not something that is distributed, and the difference in power is inescapable: for that reason we should not think of it as an imbalance or injustice *stricto sensu*. Neither is it obvious what "redressing" the difference would look like, since the final decision about whether to grant access to the information to a third party will always lie with the practitioner. (As Parker indicates, it is difficult to have an open discussion between all parties about whether to disclose information without giving away that there is something important potentially being withheld.[22]) The decision that the practitioner will have to make is analogous to the decisions that a judge would have to make in a criminal trial: that there is one person who ultimately decides on the nature, duration, and gravity of the punishment when a guilty verdict is returned means that there is a huge difference in the power held by the judge and by the defendant – but it would be perplexing to say that that arrangement needed redress. That said, the absence of structures by which the patient could get some control over what is at least ostensibly "their" information *may* be a question of how just the wider context in which the patient and practitioner operate is. To continue the judicial analogy: judges do not get to make their decisions about punishment arbitrarily, but must follow sentencing guidelines and precedents to ensure that all interested parties are justly treated – that complainants get justice, but that so does the defendant. As such, there is scope to think that there could and should be a set of publicly-scrutable guidelines that keep practitioners on track; but this is not the same as saying that there is much room for prescribed "solutions".

vi. Principles of Honour: Humility and Fidelity

So much for the Georgetown Four.

Part of the reason that some have felt the Four to be a dead weight in bioethical discussion arises from questions about whether they're the right principles to have: whether we need more, or fewer, or different ones. I shall put to one side hostility to the very idea of principlism, and accept the idea that there are certain broad principles that we might expect to see acknowledged in any recognisable account of ethics; the principles articulated as the Georgetown Four are hard to argue against without straying quite far from what would be recognised as ethics at all, and we would be puzzled by someone who claimed that, say, regard for some form justice is not a fundamental part of morality. We would be inclined to wonder whether such a person had really understood the word "morality" at all. By analogy, if somebody denied that triangles must have three sides, we would be inclined to doubt his understanding of certain basic words. But just as true statements about triangles do not exhaust geometry, there may be other principles we could consider in ethics.

Matti Häyry has provided a survey of some of the objections and alternatives to the Georgetown Four. Of particular note is his concern that there may be a cultural specificity to them: a culture in which the primacy of the individual is not central to the moral vocabulary in use may not come up with the same principles, and may understand those that are in common differently.[23] Correspondingly, the full-throated individualism of the standard model is not the only game in town – and it seems likely that a recognisably full and nuanced moral system would have to take account of agents' being alongside others. Furthermore, a moral worldview that is open to less individualistic accounts is likely to turn out to be important when we're considering how to handle genetic information, precisely because that information is by its nature transpersonal. Accordingly, I shall suggest a few more principles over the coming pages that we ought to acknowledge as important when making decisions about how to handle genetic information. These are the principles of *fidelity*, *humility*, and – in the next section – *solidarity*.

I nodded towards the principle of fidelity earlier in the book, when I suggested that breaking faith with XX, the father in the ABC case, might provide depth to his complaint when information about his diagnosis was shared with his daughter. The essence of the principle of fidelity or trust-worthiness is that commitments that we make to each other ought to be held to wherever possible. Trustworthiness is a virtue in its own right, but trust is also a necessary component of any kind of bearable existence alongside others: we have to be able to take people's word as being at least a fairly good guide to their future actions, and to be able to assure people that our word will be at least a fairly good guide to ours. If Alice has made an undertaking to Bob that she will either φ, or refrain from ψ-ing, and if he fits his behaviour to that undertaking, any instance of ψ-ing or failure to φ by Alice would be a basis for warranted complaint. If Alice is a clinician and "ψ" stands for the dissemination of information, the commitment not to ψ may very well be understood tacitly from the nature of the relation-ship; if she is Bob's aunt and "φ" stands for a promised visit to the zoo, then it will be more explicit, since taking kids to the zoo is not generally held to be a fundamental part of aunthood. In the events preceding ABC, XX had reason to believe that the staff caring for him would keep faith with him; that his expectation was defied unwittingly does not really make a differ-ence to his grounds for complaint.

Breaking faith with people may sometimes be unavoidable or unwitting; when faith is broken there may be degrees of culpability. Two persons may be at cross-purposes about what either and each can expect from their rela-tionship; and even when an expectation is well-founded, there may be per-fectly good reasons to breach a commitment. For example, suppose that someone provides a sample to a genetic databank in the expectation that it would be used in medical research, but it happens that sharing the infor-mation it yields would be useful in bringing the perpetrator of a heinous crime to justice. Here, the wrongness of the holder of that information sharing it with the police is not a given. It will be more likely to be wrong if there is an explicit promise not to share, but even then we may think that the promise ought to be broken in some circumstances. It is crucial to emphasise that the reasons to break fidelity may run afoul of countervailing reasons not to, all things considered: it may not be warranted for a trivial crime. Still, a moral reason that is overwhelmed by other moral reasons is no less of a moral reason for that. Correspondingly, that we can depart from a principle does not invalidate its status as a principle; a principle of fidelity does not tell us that it is always wrong to ψ or not to φ: only that there are *prima facie* considerations against it. We can have a good moral reason to keep faith with a person to whom we have given our word, while at the same time re-cognising that we have a competing moral reason to do what we have promised not to. Articulating the principles in play may do more to help understand the dilemma than to solve it – but understanding a dilemma is a necessary part of reaching a solution.

A principle of fidelity may also chime with a sense that one ought to be *given* access to information. Relationships may require candour that grows from trust; a failure of candour might be characterised as running contrary to a principle of keeping faith. As such, the principle of fidelity is reflected in the idea of informational privilege, and its twin demands that sharing information should be at the discretion of the referent, and that the referent should be told of – or at least not prevented from learning about – anything relevant to them. Patients may feel that the medical staff caring for them have a responsibility to give them information that is relevant to their care, and ABC might well have expected her father to tell her if he knew she was at risk from an inherited illness; in both cases, a failure to disclose could easily be characterised as a breach of fidelity. The principle may extend to third parties, too. Thus in ABC, ABC herself believed that she was owed a duty of care such that information about her father's having tested positive for Huntington's should have been given to her, and its not having been shared might well be understood as a violation of the principle of fidelity.

In chapter 2, I considered situations in which we have moral reasons to try to forget things that we have seen if we ought not to have, and at least to pretend not to have seen them if we cannot actually force amnesia, and I suggested that this kind of consideration may be important when it comes to questions of how to deal with information about a party's genome that is unwittingly shared; I linked these responsibilities with what Jane Austen called "the laws of honour".[24] A concern for fidelity would be relevant here: an accidental disclosure of information about someone may be a wrong on the part of the person who discloses it, but it makes perfect sense to think that the person to whom it is disclosed may have responsibilities based in fidelity to the referent and to the discloser in respect of it.

Equally, though, agents may also feel a kind of responsibility owed to themselves – in effect a second law of honour – to try to bury what has been unwittingly learned. This would be grounded in a feeling of personal integrity, and sensitivity to what is simply not one's proper business and that it would simply be *infra dig* to root out. This second law of honour is not captured by a principle of fidelity, since it can hold irrespective of one's relationship with other agents, or of whether there is such a relationship at all. For example, a paparazzo who declines a job because he decides that it is just too sordid is not acting out of any sense of fidelity. What is in play here is a related but much more "inward-looking" principle that I shall call the principle of humility.

Part of the idea here is that whatever one's reasons to access information, the recognition that there are competing interests at stake gives one a moral reason to check one's enthusiasm for them: to adopt an attitude of humility towards one's own claims in the light of others'. However, there is another part of it that does not depend on the presence of competing claims but much more directly on a willingness to step back from, and take a more considered view of, one's presently-occurring desires – in essence, asking oneself whether this or that is *really* what one wants or needs to do, notwithstanding the reasons one has to do it. Put another way, it concerns the virtue of knowing when not to impose oneself on the world, or when not to take up too much moral space.

Insofar as that to breach privacy is, *per* the definition I offered in chapter 2, to bring into the light something that would not otherwise have been there, the principle of humility fits well into models of maintaining privacy: it counsels us that there may be times when it would be desirable or admirable to hold back from accessing information to which we *could*, but presently do not, have access. It is the antithesis to a principle of nosiness, and an appeal to something like a principle of humility helps explain what is morally troubling about nosiness. The principle of humility helps explain the argument that the Access to Self account of privacy rights comes "too late", and it also speaks to the distinction between seeing and watching, or (as I considered in chapter 5) seeing and prying. A principle of humility nudges us away from putting ourselves in a position in which we are likely to expose ourselves to what is unbecoming – and it does so not because of the person whom we have seen, but because of ourselves. And we can see here an answer to the question I posed in chapter 5 about whether prying is wrong because it violates rights, or whether rights are violated because of the wrongness of prying: a right being something that one ascribes to agents at the conclusion of a process of moral reasoning, we can say that rights are violated because of the disapprobation within which we hold prying, which violates the principle of humility.

However, saying that we have moral reasons to try to put to one side of things that we have seen but ought not to have is to risk begging the question, since it smuggles in a claim that these are things that we ought not to have seen in the first place; absent that, the moral reasons seem to vanish. And while there may be something admirable about one party in a conflict about access to information adopting an attitude of humility and choosing not to press the case, it does not seem to be more than supererogatory. Whereas something like a concern for justice (whatever that turns out to be or to require) looks as though it is built in to thinking clearly about ethics in any sense, and one can require that people behave in a way dictated by justice, an attitude of humility works differently. Humility is not an axiom of morality; one cannot require humility of people in the same way that one can require justice, and while a just distribution of some good is still just even if it is distributed under duress, mandatory humility is pantomime humility. As such, while something like a principle of humility would be *found* in a fully-rounded common morality, it will not be central; it is unlikely to be a decisive decisionmaking tool when two parties have conflicting claims from which neither is willing to back down. Emma could not impose humility on Gerry or Terry.

Yet the risk of begging the question is not a certainty. When we say that information ought not to have been shared, we may simply mean that it was a mishap. Granted this, humility may be recommended on its own merits. Still, that is compatible with saying that it is one principle that has to fight for space with others. Fitting it with the wider ethical picture I am painting, we would say that one's reasons to act according to a principle of humility obtain only to the extent that that is the most pressing consideration at a given time. Whether we are ever in such a time is an open question. But even if we are not, we can still acknowledge humility as a virtue, or as providing a reason for action (or inaction). And it does seem reasonable to think that a principle of humility may come into play in some circumstances. For example, suppose that Gerry had made it known that he was going to have his genome sequenced, and family members had expressed qualms about it. If Gerry's desire to know about his genome is based on a morally weighty concern, Terry's claims about privacy could perhaps be set aside; but when the motivation is idle curiosity, a principle of humility may give him pause, and will do so even without Terry having to have a clear and bankable *ab initio* right to privacy. A principle of humility would not *mandate* a self-denying ordinance – but it would give Gerry a reason to hesitate, and such hesitation may be admirable. On the other hand, we would presumably also want to be sure that this really was humility, rather than something more like self-abasement, which we would not want to endorse as a principle. And a principle of humility would give Terry a reason not to veto Gerry's test that would have to be balanced with the reasons for his qualms.

Equally, XX's refusal to share his genetic information with ABC in order to nudge her reproductive decisions looks – as I have argued – like an instance of his failure to treat her as a moral equal, and like a misappropriation of power and therefore unjust; but it could just as well be characterised as an over-estimation of the importance of his own desires. This amounts to a failure of humility. The difference between a principle of humility and a principle of justice in something like the ABC case is that the principle of justice involves seeing the world disinterestedly, from a god's-eye perspective. Humility makes no demand for disinterest. And as such, it is similar to one proposed addition to the Georgetown Four that has garnered quite a lot of attention: the idea of solidarity.

vii. The Principle of Solidarity

Inasmuch as that solidarity speaks directly to the relationships between people, and that disputes and problems about the control of and access to genetic information arise (I have argued) substantially because such information is not "confined" to one person at a time – and can only really be understood once that is taken into account – one may wonder whether solidarity would be important in the context of questions about genetics.

Solidarity has been defined in numerous ways, though the similarities between accounts should allow us to get a flavour of the concept. For Häyry, solidarity "is often portrayed as the European counterpart of justice", and it

> is related to, but should not be confused with, the liberal and utilitarian accounts of fairness and equality. Liberals usually emphasize the protection of the rights of individuals, and utilitarians focus on the equal consideration of, and equal respect for, the needs and interests of individuals. In both models, the state is seen as a primary force behind the coercive organization of social life. Solidarity, in contrast, is in European debates linked with communities rather than official state functions, voluntary rather than enforced activities, spontaneous rather than organized events, and reciprocal rather than contractual exchanges.[25]

I would add to this the thought that, whereas justice is a "cognitive" virtue, understood in terms of beliefs about what is fair or rightful, solidarity is "non-cognitive": it draws from our relationships with people or groups of people, but it does not offer propositions that lend themselves to belief or disbelief. In this, it resembles Gilligan's concept of "care".[26] Elsewhere, Häyry points out that treating people differently from others based on physical characteristics may undermine solidarity,[27] and this point clearly echoes the classic Aristotelian account of justice.[28] So far so good; but saying that it is related to justice without being quite the same this is not enough to nail down quite what solidarity *is*.

The work of Prainsack and Buyx adds significantly to that matter. Their 2012 paper notes an increasing number of appeals to solidarity in the bioethical literature, and attempts to discern what is being talked about and its importance. They identify three tiers to solidarity, the first of which is the individual. On this tier, "solidarity comprises manifestations of the willingness to carry costs to assist others with whom a person recognizes sameness or similarity in at least one relevant respect".[29] This definition is reflected in their expanded 2017 account of solidarity, which offers as a working definition of solidarity that it "is an enacted commitment to carry 'costs' (financial, social, emotional or otherwise) to assist others with whom a person or persons recognise similarity in a relevant respect".[30]

A willingness to act, potentially thereby incurring real or symbolic costs, is important when it comes to distinguishing solidarity from sympathy – an ability and willingness to take on another person's emotional state as one's own – and empathy – a willingness to project oneself into that other person's state. Someone who is sitting on a delayed aeroplane next to a passenger who is worried she will miss her connection may be sympathetic but do nothing; someone thinking about what it would be like to be in that predicament may be emphathising, but be unable to do anything or have anything to do; she will only be showing solidarity if she does something like lend her companion her mobile phone to make arrangements when they land.[31]

The second tier of solidarity arises when

> a particular solidaristic practice at the inter-personal level becomes so normal that it is more widely seen as 'good conduct' in a given situation, [and] can solidify into forms of institutionalisation. This is the case, for example, with respect to self-help groups that practise more institutionalised solidarity. On this tier, solidarity can be described as *manifestations of a collective commitment to carry costs to assist others (who are all linked by means of a shared situation or cause)*. This is the second and arguably most prominent tier of solidarity. People who share a situation typically share certain risks or positive goals which emerge out of, or define, that situation.[32]

The 2017 recapitulation of their account suggests that second-tier solidarity rests on both a "collective" and a "shared" commitment to carry costs to assist others.[33] It is possible that these are not quite the same; but either way, they feed through to a third tier of solidarity in which the values and principles arising at the second tier "manifest themselves in contractual or other legal norms":

> Examples are welfare state and welfare society arrangements, or legal arrangements underpinning publicly funded healthcare systems[.] Such legal and contractual arrangements are highly institutionalized enactments of carrying costs to assist others one recognizes sameness with, for example by collecting taxes from the population to fund the services provided to those in need of healthcare.[34]

Tiers two and three in this schema are plainly derivative of the first: tier two collective commitment presupposes some kind of basic solidarity that explains the origin of the collective that makes commitments. What matters for my purposes is the idea that solidarity at its core differs from empathy because it is not simply a matter of being able to put oneself in others' shoes: it is (at the very least) a disposition to share their burden; and it differs from justice because it makes no appeal to and is not limited by any demands of fairness when it comes to taking on the burden. Finally, a willingness to take on costs is important when it comes from distinguishing solidarity from humility. The similarity between the two lies in the way that they both involve a kind of making-way for the another; but whereas humility does so by enjoining us to make way in the sense of getting out of that other's path, solidarity enjoins us to make way in the more radicalised sense of helping them to clear that path in the first place.

One question would concern what counts in the first tier as the "relevant aspect" in which one sees oneself as similar to the other. For Prainsack and Buyx, this is a crucial part of their understanding of the concept: solidarity is context-specific. Similarity in a relevant respect is determined by the situation in which agents find themselves, and so solidarity must be defined in terms of whatever it is that binds people together at a given moment.[35] If there are several morally-relevant similarities, they continue, this may mean that solidarity deepens into something more, like friendship. This suggests that there is a kind of "upper limit" to solidarity: "[t]he better people know each other", they argue, "the more likely they are to be bound together by stronger bonds than solidarity" – and the stronger and closer the emotional bonds between people, the more solidarity between them may become "redundant".[36] Solidarity, then (if Prainsack and Buyx are right), occupies the space between mutual indifference and friendship, and in a way it keeps others at a distance.

Prainsak and Buyx acknowledge the work of Darryl Gunson, for whom a basic definition of solidarity is that it "consists in the willingness to take the perspective of others seriously and *to act in support of it*".[37] This definition admits of further refinement, though, as Gunson distinguishes between what he calls *strong* and *weak* solidarity. Weak solidarity is "the willingness to take the perspective of others seriously"; strong solidarity is "the aspect of solidarity that emphasizes support for specific goals or political causes. It is the solidarity of action that is central to many of the paradigmatic uses of the term".[38] As such, though he does not say as much, the implication of Gunson's position is that weak solidarity is very weak indeed, perhaps devolving to sympathy or humility. Genuine – strong – solidarity is motivationally ert,[39] and to stand in a solidaristic relationship with someone would, by definition, be to have a reason to act (although what that action is would remain undetermined). On the other hand, solidarity on Gunson's understanding is not quite so emotionally demanding as that in some other accounts: even strong solidarity is compatible with disinterest. As such, it would appear that Mr Spock may be capable of solidarity, even if he is not capable of empathy. (From this, one may surmise that weak solidarity would be motivationally inert compared even to sympathy or empathy, since it contains neither a conceptually-required requirement to act, nor the emotional impetus of sympathy or empathy.)

viii. The Uses of Solidarity

How might this be of any use here?

Solidarity is interpersonal by its nature, and this is why it appears to be worth bringing to the table when considering relationships between agents insofar as that they hold things such as genomes or an interest in genetic information in common.[40] It requires taking into account the existence and the needs of at least one other person, and adopting that existence and those needs as a determining factor when it comes to moral decisionmaking. Solidarity may beget a kind of beneficence, since a recognition of the other's needs and interests may be hard to separate from the recognition of a moral reason to act in a way that would alleviate those needs and further those interests. But it is not reducible to beneficence, which can have a slightly patrician sense to it that is absent from solidarity. Furthermore, beneficence implies that the beneficent person is in a position to bestow benefit; yet it is possible for, say, a penniless person to have at least a sense of weak solidarity with a millionaire traduced in the press, especially if that millionaire is being traduced for standing in defence of what the poor person sees as a noble cause. (Prainsack and Buyx are correct to suggest that solidarity will generally be expressed by the less vulnerable towards the more[41]; but "generally" is not "necessarily", and the less vulnerable are less likely to find themselves in positions that attract solidarity in the first place.)

Although solidarity requires a kind of keeping-apart between agents, its interpersonal aspect militates against competitiveness between those agents in respect of the *locus* of their solidarity. And this is well-fitted to a view of human affairs in which agents are fundamentally interconnected. It appears to follow from this that a principle of solidarity may be important to keep in mind when it comes to the handling of genetic information and data, since that is, *ex hypothesi*, not confined to just the one person at a time. "[I]f we hold that people are intrinsically connected to each other", suggest Prainsack and Buyx, "then it is farfetched to assume that the collection, sharing, discussion and use of personal health information would regularly be a solipsistic and self-centred activity".[42]

And what is less centred on any given self than genetic information? As Prainsack and Buyx point out,

> [g]enetic data always relate to others, not only because they can disclose information about biological relatives of the person who they came from, but also because people often want to know their 'genetic risk' out of concern for others: because they are convinced that having this information will help them with their reproductive decision-making or because they want to share this information with their friends or families.[43]

There seems to be plenty of reason to think that solidarity would be a relevant consideration when it comes to decisions about genetic information.

Still, things may not be completely straightforward. Though the promise of solidarity is that it is non-competitive, the problem with genetic information is that the interests that agents have over control of genetic information frequently *are* competitive. By and large, the more control over genetic information one person has, the less another has. So although solidarity does imply a willingness to take on some of the costs of assisting others, it is not obvious how applicable this idea is in the sort of context we are considering here. This is not least because to take on some cost as part of standing in solidarity with another must surely be different from relinquishing one's interests altogether: solidarity in the face of direct conflicts of interest is not possible. One could stand in solidarity with someone when some or even most of one's interests conflict with them (hence Manchester United fans may be intensely competitive with Liverpool fans in almost all respects, but stand in solidarity with them in respect of the Hillsborough disaster), and this is often implicit in the idea that solidarity implies the willingness to make a sacrifice (hence someone might support a tax rate rise that is not in their direct interest, because they think that social services for the least-well-off should be better funded). But standing in putative solidarity with a person *in respect of the thing over which one's interests conflict* is simply to cede the field, and thereby to dissolve the conflict of interests. It is tempting to think that one could still express solidarity with the person with whom one finds oneself in competition insofar as that one would be moved by their disappointment were one's preferred outcome to be realised: an athlete may be moved by the sight of a long-term rival falling. But I think that that is probably sympathy or empathy, rather than solidarity. For this reason, it's not obvious how solidarity would have much of a role in explaining the moral dimensions of any dispute between Kerry and Perry or between Gerry and Terry.

A second difficulty with expecting too much from solidarity when trying to adjudicate on disputes arising from the control of genetic information is that, like the principle of humility, solidarity has little normative force; it is non-cognitive, which means that it would be hard to show that a statement like "this is insufficiently solidaristic" could ever be true. Equally, it is not clear how someone could be mistaken in their assessment of how to demonstrate solidarity, beyond there being a point at which other competent users of the language would simply be able to say that the word is or is not appropriate as a descriptor of their actions. And it is certainly not enforceable. Even if Perry were to try to make the case that Kerry ought to share information about her genome out of solidarity, then presumably Kerry would be able to make the case that Perry should relinquish her claim on the basis of exactly the same principle. We would get nowhere.

A characteristic of three of the Georgetown Four principles is that they describe attitudes the failure to act upon which would be blameable: we could blame someone for maleficence, for failing to take sufficient regard of agents' autonomy, or for injustice, on the basis that they had fallen short of some fairly fundamental standard of proper behaviour. The principle of beneficence is a bit of an outlier here, since it is less obvious that a person who thinks that the world is good enough in some respect would have fallen short by not improving it. In this respect, it behaves in the same sort of way as the principle of solidarity (and the principle of humility): if someone does not behave in a particularly solidaristic manner, this does not mean that they are undermining anyone else's interests; and, as such, it is not obvious that there would be any particular grounds to find positive wrongdoing so much as to diagnose a character flaw. Accordingly, though we might think that it is a good or honourable thing to allow one's genetic information to be shared for the sake of others' good under at least some circumstances, where we go from there may not be self-evident: if they prefer to take what measures they can to keep it to themselves, then that is more or less the whole story. Solidarity requires an agent to choose it for its own sake.[44] It is not something that can be required.

Neither is it likely that a principle of solidarity would help explain what is going on when a healthcare professional is trying to decide whether or not to disclose a piece of sensitive information, genetic or otherwise. After all, there is no sacrifice from the decisionmaker involved here – no willingness to take on a burden for the sake of a perceived good. At most, a medic might risk professional censure for having breached expectations about privacy and confidentiality; but while it may look as though this could count as the sacrifice that is implicit in solidaristic action, that would not really be tenable, since what is sacrificed really is the autonomy of the patient whose decision is nullified. Disciplinary action is a sequela to *that*.

This is not to say that solidarity is irrelevant. There may be considerations of solidarity in play when it comes to decisions about whether, and under what conditions, to share genetic data, or (perhaps more particularly) genetic information, and allow it to be shared. In particular, something along the lines of tier-three solidarity may be relevant when we are thinking about the attitude we should take to biosamples being accessed in the name of criminal justice or some other aspect of the public good. We could not derive from an appeal to solidarity any claim that someone *ought* to allow their information to be used. However, a sense of solidarity may explain their sense that they would allow it even if we think that it would not be mandatory all things considered; correspondingly, a person may interrogate her own sense of solidarity and its contours to reach a decision about whether to accede to any other request for access to information or data-sharing. A person may, on the basis of introspection about her own commitments, decide that she ought to allow information about her genome to be shared and used in a particular way, even though that is perhaps not something that she would intuitively have allowed. This sort of self-discovery is entirely of a piece with the fairly normal process of working out exactly what one's commitments are, how they mesh together, and what they require of us.

Such reasoning about our own commitments is likely to be fairly complicated. If we allow that solidarity is a relevant attitude or consideration when solving problems raised by genetic information, it may still pull an agent in more than one direction. Suppose that Kerry is persuaded that solidarity with those whom Perry represents gives her a reason to disclose genetic information about herself. In doing so, she will also disclose information about her sister Sherry, and her daughter Cherry. But one might perfectly reasonably expect Kerry to have some relationship with them that is characterised by, among other things, a sense of solidarity; and this could plausibly give her a reason *not* to disclose. How, then, are we to decide what practical effect an appeal to solidarity would have? A similar question might be raised in respect of Gerry and Terry's extended family; it might not only be Gerry who wants to know about his genome: he might want to know about it because of a concern about his blood relatives, offspring, or merely potential offspring, and this motive may involve something appreciably like solidarity.

One might try to weigh up the consequences of disclosure or non-disclosure – but this would mean abandoning solidarity in favour of a fairly basic utilitarianism; and if we are willing to do that, then why not cut to the chase and be utilitarians right from the start? The consequences of a decision are almost certainly morally salient; but a fully rich account of moral decision-making would consider the importance of those consequences among other things: essentially, the principles of beneficence and nonmaleficence would have to be considered alongside other principles.

Finally, it is worth keeping in mind that solidarity need not be of direct import to Kerry and Perry (or Gerry and Terry, for that matter); and Prainsack and Buyx's second and third tiers of solidarity explain why. Recall that one of the major concerns surrounding the idea that Kerry might be forced to share her information was that she would thereby be disenfranchised from some goods – certain kinds of insurance may be one such lost good, and potentially (and much more seriously) loss of access to healthcare might be a life-shortening consequence of that. However, third-tier solidarity is treated explicitly as bringing with it goods such as welfare states' public health systems.[45] Tier-one solidarity between Kerry and Perry may not offer all that much in terms of deciding who should have access to what information and under what terms; and it might be that seeing the problem as nothing more than one of competing claims about rights or interests would force us to admit that Kerry should surrender her information. There is no law of interpersonal relations that says that they must be resolved in a way that is to everyone's satisfaction all the time: some bullets just have to be bitten. But neither is there a law that says that we must keep our analysis at the interpersonal level. If we accept that genomes are suprapersonal we already have an example of being able to think at a much higher level. And the state is a suprapersonal institution. Of course, from the fact that A and B are stipulated both to have some predicate in common, it does not follow that one will tell us much about the other. Nevertheless, it does not seem as though it would be scandalously impertinent to think that the state, either through law or through delegated authority of some sort, might be the kind of thing that could plausibly help solve problems generated by interpersonal relationships. And it can do so in the name of solidarity. Bluntly, a state's failure to ensure that all its denizens have access to at least basic goods can be seen as a failure of tier-three solidarity; its failure to ensure that one's genetic inheritance is irrelevant on this front can be seen in the same way. As we have seen, this may help set the tone of the Kerry and Perry debate.

ix. Bringing Privacy Back

In the chapters leading up to this, I have made the case that the idea of genetic privacy is too slippery to be something that we can expect as a matter of right. A reductionist account might suggest that this is too bad for the idea of a right to genetic privacy: it is something in which we as a culture should stop believing, roughly as we stopped believing in ontologically distinct minds.

But people do talk about their minds without difficulty and without any abiding commitment to dualism. In fact, using "mind" as a shorthand for "whatever it is that thinks, feels, experiences, and so on" makes many conversations much more manageable. Terms and practices can have a perfectly useful and legitimate place in everyday discourse and behaviour even when nobody takes them particularly seriously in their own right, or even when a word has no clear reference. And this, I would aver, is what is going on when we talk about rights to genetic privacy. We do not have to treat such a right as a *datum* in discussions about who should have access to what and on what terms. Rather, our statement that Terry has no right to privacy is an articulation of the conclusions we have reached based on a consideration of the competing reasons that he and Gerry have to control access to the information in their shared genome. When we claim that Kerry's right to privacy means that she need not share genetic information with Perry the insurer, we are saying that the principles in play shake out that way.

We are using a claim about rights to describe positions in a process of moral deliberation, rather than as factors to consider in that deliberation. We are ascribing rights, some of which will be generalisable (for example, if we are considering what to put into a policy about the entitlement of the police to examine information held by direct-to-consumer genetic test providers), and some of which will have currency only in the context of a given relationship.

Put another way, we can say that a person has a right to access information just when, all things considered, it is reasonable that they should be able to do so. Conversely, a person can expect privacy to be maintained when others have no reasonable justification for accessing information; and that expectation amounts to a right when those others have compelling moral reasons *not* to access it. (This claim is something like Marmor's.[46]) Remember in this context that privacy is the default state for genetic information. Either way, though, the language of rights still has a place in our conversations, even if it does not denote quite what we might have thought it denoted.

These conversations will be informed by a number of competing principles, and there need be no *a priori* way to compare and align them. Not all will be relevant in all cases, and not all will have the same heft from one case to another; there may be other principles that we can and should consider, too – for example, Amy Cohen has suggested that concocting something like a right to privacy may be desirable for the sake of facilitating "fundamental public policy goals relating to liberal democratic citizenship, innovation, and human flourishing".[47] I have suggested, though, that justice will be of singular importance, because questions about access to and control over genetic information will almost always become questions about what degree of access should be allocated to whom, and who should cede what control to whom. "The just" will be understood as the distribution of control over that information that is most satisfactory all things considered. With unconfined information, it probably could not be otherwise, and we will always in some sense be having to think about preferred allocations of control over information, since what we do with information is not simply about one person at a time, and "informational privilege" turns out to be an illusion. As such, normative questions can be understood by considering possible allocations of control, and deciding whether the word "just" could be applied, and how close a fit it would be, granted the role that the word plays in the language.

Vitally importantly, every participant in a debate about what rights to ascribe to whom will have their own intuitions about what weight to give each of those principles. It will not always be easy to determine in advance what rights a person really does have – but there would, nevertheless, still be in principle (as it were) an answer or (at most) a small number of equally plausible answers to be had, even if discerning them would be a Herculean task. Nevertheless, weighing principles against each other ought still to be possible – and at the very least, a process of public reasoning could help us evaluate certain courses of action.

For example, we could probably discard the idea that Kerry should have to surrender all control of information about her genome to Perry, because that would not be a just allocation; but we could also (perhaps with a bit more soul-searching) discard the idea that there would never be a situation in which she may keep all the control for herself. Somewhere between those poles, an optimal distribution will be found. The just allocation of control would be homed in on by considering whether the word "just" fits scenario 1 or 2 better; justice as a principle could then be weighed in light of other principles that would have been subject to a similar process of public reasoning (for example, to determine whether a proposed course of action shows humility or self-denial, solidarity or meretriciousness).

The best, and right, course of action will depend on what virtues and principles we identify as being relevant, and how they play against each other, and on the external circumstances. In a country with little to no public provision of healthcare, we may want to say that Perry will on balance have a less strong claim to access information than Kerry has to withhold it; this amounts to saying that Perry's rights may be much more restricted than they would be in a country in which Kerry's access to other goods is not materially affected by how easily she can buy affordable insurance. Alternatively, allowing that Perry has a case to be given a right of access to at least some of Kerry's genetic information for a certain purpose is one thing; but we would also likely discard the idea that that right applies to all genetic information. For example, if Perry is selling motor insurance, Kerry's risk of breast cancer would be irrelevant, and there would therefore be no reason for Perry to be provided with it. Such provision would be gratuitous, and for Perry to seek it would be indicative of a violation of the principle of humility. Likewise, we would probably want to discard the possibility that Perry may sell information about Kerry's genome on to third parties, or to trawl existing databases in order to spot and exploit marketing opportunities – though we may be more circumspect about discarding the possibility that she may pass it on to detectives searching for a murderer.

In practice, and given the limitations of human minds and the open texture of moral language, it is unlikely that there would be in every case certainty about either the precise weight to give to a given principle, or the precise way in which it interacts with other salient principles. Therefore, although we may expect that it would be possible to eliminate most notionally possible attributions of rights in respect of genetic information – to say that a given distribution of control is just or unjust, and whether a given claim can properly be said to reflect this or that principle – it will always be possible that there could be several reasonable attributions, and perhaps a couple between which there is no definitive difference to be drawn and we are in a situation of genuine equipoise: it would actually be surprising if there were not sometimes situations in which we find ourselves caught between two opposing views, each of which has merits and demerits. Should there be two competing courses of action apparent to us, we could at the very least comfort ourselves with the thought that, whichever we choose, it will not have been the wrong one.

If all this sounds rather vague, I have no defence – but neither would I attempt one: it does not seem to me to be a failure of an account of ethics that there is no clear and pre-defined set of answers that we can apply quickly and easily to the very complicated world we inhabit. In fact, it is a strength rather than a weakness of a moral theory that it can recognise that there is such a thing as a genuine dilemma. We should aim to talk about agents and their rights in respect of genetic information in terms of their relationships. Rights are not *data* in such talk: they are things we can deduce as products of relationships between people and those people's projects; and as such, it is possible that any rights will be as various and as protean as the relationships between people. The point-centres of force to which Mackie referred are not static; the interplay of forces, and which holds sway at a given time and in a given place, will move.

The difficulty lies in enforcement of the outcomes of moral deliberation. In the next and final chapter, I shall attempt to say a little more about how the principles outlined here may play out in some real-world contexts and in law and policy.

Notes

1 Jeremy Waldron notes that rights "do not provide reasons for acting, at least not for the people who have them" ("A Right to Do Wrong" *Ethics* 92[1] (1981), p 28). The second clause is the important one here. Alice's right to have a nice hot bath does not give her a reason to have one; but her right that Bob should run it for her when she tells him to gives him a reason to run it should she tell him to.

2 Mackie, JL, "Can There Be a Right-Based Moral Theory?" *Midwest Studies in Philosophy* 3[1] (1978), p 351.

3 *ibid*, p 356.

4 *ibid*, p 356.

5 *ibid*, p 356.

6 *vide* Dworkin, R, "Is There a Right to Pornography?" *Oxford Journal of Legal Studies* 1[2] (1981), p 200; *Taking Rights Seriously* (London: Bloomsbury, 2013), *passim*.

7 Nozick, R, *Anarchy, State, and Utopia* (New York: Basic Books, 1974), pp 29ff.

8 Dworkin, *op cit* (2013) p 118.

9 Mills, K, "Consent and the Right to Privacy", *Journal of Applied Philosophy* 39[4] (2022), p 731 (slightly modified).

10 *vide* Graeber, D, *Debt: The First 5000 Years* (Brooklyn, NY: Melville House, 2012), chs 1–4; Martin, F, *Money: The Unauthorised Biography* (London: Vintage, 2014).

11 I restrict my discussion to putative rights of genetic privacy; the shape of the argument may extend to other rights, or even to all rights – but showing that it does would require an argument that I have no desire to construct at the moment.

12 Beauchamp, T, & Childress, J, *Principles of Biomedical Ethics, 7th Edition* (New York: Oxford UP, 2013).

13 Gillon, R, "Ethics Needs Principles – Four Can Encompass the Rest – and Respect for Autonomy Should Be 'First among Equals'", *Journal of Medical Ethics* 28[5] (2003), *passim*.

14 Beauchamp & Childress, *op cit*, p ix.

15 Beauchamp & Childress, *op cit*, p 152.

16 Beauchamp & Childress, *op cit*, pp 202–203.

17 Rawls, 1999, *passim*.

18 Rawls, J, *A Theory of Justice* (Oxford: Oxford UP, 1999), §46 and *passim*.

19 Rawls, J, *Political Liberalism* (New York: Columbia UP, 2005), p 180 and *passim*.

20 *ibid*, p 181 (slightly modified).

21 Hoven, J van den, & Rooksby, E, "Distributive Justice and the Value of Information: A (Broadly) Rawlsian Approach", in Hoven, J van den, & Weckert, J (eds), *Information Technology and Moral Philosophy* (Cambridge: Cambridge UP, 2008), p 384 and *passim*.

22 Parker, M, "Genetics and the Interpersonal Elaboration of Ethics", *Theoretical Medicine and Bioethics* 22[5] (2001), *passim*.

23 Häyry, M, "European Values in Bioethics: Why, What, and How to Be Used?" *Theoretical Medicine and Bioethics* 24[3] (2003), *passim*; Häyry, M, "Precaution and Solidarity", *Cambridge Quarterly of Healthcare Ethics* 14[2] (2005), p 199; but cf Beachamp & Childress, *op cit*, p ix.

24 Austen, J, *Persuasion* (London: Penguin, 1985), p 210.

25 Häyry, *op cit* (2003), p 206; cf Häyry, *op cit* (2005), esp p 204.

26 Gilligan, C, *In a Different Voice* (Cambridge, Mass: Harvard UP, 1993), *passim*.

27 Häyry, M, *Rationality and the Genetic Challenge* (Cambridge: Cambridge UP, 2010), p 6.

28 Aristotle, *The Politics* (London: Penguin, 1992), 1280a7ff; Aristotle, *The Nichomachean Ethics* (Oxford: Oxford UP, 2009), 1131a10ff.

29 Prainsack, B, & Buyx, A, "Solidarity in Contemporary Bioethics – towards a New Approach", *Bioethics* 26[7] (2012), p 346.

30 Prainsack, B, & Buyx, A, *Solidarity in Biomedicine and Beyond* (Cambridge: Cambridge UP, 2017), p 52.
31 Prainsack and Buyx, *op cit* (2012), p 347.
32 *ibid*, p 347.
33 Prainsack & Buyx, *op cit* (2017), p 55.
34 Prainsack and Buyx, *op cit* (2012), p 347.
35 Prainsack & Buyx, *op cit* (2017), p 52.
36 Prainsack & Buyx, *op cit* (2017), p 60.
37 Gunson, D, "Solidarity and the Universal Declaration on Bioethics and Human Rights", *Journal of Medicine and Philosophy* 34[3] (2009), p 247.
38 *ibid*.
39 What I cannot avoid calling *ertia* is the opposite of inertia; correspondingly, something's being ert is the opposite of its being inert.
40 Relatedly, see Gilbar, R, "Communicating Genetic Information in the Family: The Familial Relationship as the Forgotten Factor", *Journal of Medical Ethics* 33[7] (2007), *passim*.
41 Prainsack and Buyx, *op cit* (2012), p 347.
42 Prainsack & Buyx, *op cit* (2017), p 132.
43 *ibid*, p 132.
44 *ibid*, p 58.
45 *ibid*, p 56.
46 Marmor, A, "What Is the Right to Privacy?" *Philosophy and Public Affairs* 43[1] (2015), *passim*.
47 Cohen, A, "What Privacy Is For", *Harvard Law Review* 126[7] (2013), p 1928.

8 Reinvention and Regulation

i. Recapitulation

In chapter 1 of this book, I outlined a "standard model" of bioethics, and sketched out how it tends to be applied to questions of how to control information. I also suggested that, in respect of genetic information, there may be concerns about the neat applicability of the standard model. In chapter 3, I tried to put some flesh on those bones, showing that a naïve application of the standard model when it comes to genetic privacy can get us into strange and messy situations that we would want to avoid. The Gerry and Terry problem outlined there is, admittedly, painted in unrealistically bright primary colours – but it does serve a purpose, which is to illustrate how claims about privacy can turn into much more perplexing claims involving what I identified as secrecy and taboo. And it turns out (I argued) that the theoretical bases for a putative right to privacy are likely to struggle in respect of genetic information; and if I am correct on this, then the perplexities of things like the Gerry and Terry case ought not to surprise us.

Even if there were a theoretically sound basis for the concept of a right to genetic privacy, we would still have moral reasons to think that one ought to share at least some genetic information at least some of the time. But if that is correct, what has happened to the right? What sense can we make of a right to privacy that one ought sometimes to relinquish? Or, to put it another way, of a right to privacy that can be trumped by another's (putative) right to access?

What is crucial, I think, is interests. On the basis of a full account of whose interests are engaged in a given situation, and in what way they are engaged, we can hope to be able to talk about a right to genetic privacy not as a *datum* in moral debate, but as its outcome. These rights are not things that we have *ab initio*, but are things that are derived. From this claim, though, a number of questions appears on the horizon. If this is the case in respect of *privacy*, what about the related concept of *confidentiality* as a right, too? And why only genetic information?

It is answers to questions such as these that I shall outline in this chapter. I shall also apply the analysis offered over the last pages to a few real-world problems: questions that arise in respect of direct-to-consumer genetic

DOI: 10.4324/9781003312512-12

testing, of third-party (primarily insurer and police) access to genetic data-banks, and of clinicians' duties to inform and warn. I shall also look at what the argument developed so far might imply for law and professional regulation, arguing that both already have the resources to deal with the slightly open-ended account of rights to genetic privacy that I have been outlining. That rights are taken from the negotiating-table, rather than brought to them, is not all that important. The alternative to writing a law or a regulation for every possible situation is to put in place laws and regulations that can tolerate, or that mandate, judgements that if not quite made case-by-case, are at least sensitive to the circumstances at hand.

But before getting to that, I think I need to face down a couple of possible objections.

ii. The Language of Rights

The obvious objection to the picture I have tried to paint so far is that it commits us to putting a great deal of effort into saying not very much at all, and that in doing so it may actually erode a fair amount of what we think valuable. The everyday language of rights *does* articulate something that we can bring to the table that will act as an *ab initio* curb on the kinds of things that other persons may do to us and that we may do to them. That our everyday language might stand in need of revision is not all that big a deal, of course: the word "phlogiston" had a place and pulled its weight in scientific discourse until it didn't, and the fact that it did was not a reason to strive to keep it. However, the familiar way in which rights-talk is deployed does have characteristics that we might want to preserve. Not the least of these is that it makes interactions between agents morally predictable, which seems like a desirable sort of thing; to deny that rights are the *data* of moral debate is to imperil that. The idea that I have a right to life means that, right from the start of any discussion about what you may do to me, there is at least one thing that you may not; and the same would apply to any other right. A right to privacy over one's genetic data means that each of us knows where we stand. Again, this is not in itself a reason to believe in such a right as a *datum* of debate; but it does give us reasons to endorse it as a given. There does seem to be potentially quite a lot at stake, and we might be wary of destabilising an edifice that gives us quite a lot of the moral protections and security that we tend to want. I shall return to the predictability point in a little while.

Finally, the language of rights as we are used to it seems to provide a good way to sustain quite a lot of other moral concepts. One of these is the concept of forgiveness. Suppose that I have a right to φ that you have violated in some way. In most cases, we would want to say that you should be censured; but censure is not always appropriate. If I pose some direct threat to your life, your killing me, or acting in some way that would predictably precipitate my demise, ought not to attract censure should that have been the only way for you to protect your own right to life. It might even be that things other than your right to life could generate apparently serious challenges to my own: there may be cultural artefacts that we could hold to be so valuable that killing in order to preserve them begins to look like a plausible moral option. Or if I am a baker and you are on the brink of starvation, stealing a loaf from me may be defensible. Yet contrary to appearances, the argument goes, examples like this would not mean that my right to life or to property was forfeit; and this is because your actions would not be *permissible* so much as *forgivable* – and forgiveness implies impermissibility. On this view, moral dilemmas can be generated by genuine and thoroughgoing conflicts of rights.

Relatedly, consider the hackneyed thought-experiment in which trapped cavers are trapped in a cavern and their only means of escape involves killing one of their number.[1] In this sort of case, we might think that the cavers (or their insurers, at the very least) owe the estate of the dead man some form of compensation, and that those whose survival was bought by homicide ought at the very least to regret deeply what they ended up having to do; and we would be horrified if we thought that those survivors made the decision lightly. Yet we might think that there would be no cause for regret had there been no wrong; and the wrong would be easiest to account for by assuming that there had been a right violated.[2] Likewise, we may think that this is the sort of situation in which the law ought at least to take an interest, even if it decides that it would not serve the public interest to prosecute, or to impose as heavy a sentence as it might in other circumstances. And there are cases in which the law's behaviour could be explained in this way. In *R v Dudley and Stephens*, two castaways who had killed and eaten the cabin-boy Parker in the belief that this was a prerequisite of their survival were found guilty of murder: it was held that necessity was no defence.[3] Nevertheless, a recommendation of mercy was made, and they served what amounted to a token sentence. Here, we might think that the best explanation of this is precisely that Parker had certain rights and that the law ought to have acted in recognition of Dudley and Stephens's having violated those rights, even if the proper level of punishment was more-or-less notional because they also had a right to life that they could not have been required to surrender.

At other times, an agent may not have to choose between his own or someone else's rights; he may have to choose between two others'. For example, as in the *Tarasoff* case, we might think that a person has a right to be warned of a serious threat, even if that means infringing on another person's right to confidentiality. This is slightly different from the cases in the last paragraph, because deciding to warn would not so obviously require compensation or contrition. But, once again, the basic situation would be one in which the proper consideration of the conflicting rights in play would be a part of deciding what to do. Each relevant right would be a *datum* in the overall moral evaluation of the situation – something that each party had, and which had to be weighed against the other party's rights.

But the picture I have presented here is not like this. My claim has not been that there is a right to privacy concerning genetic information that we

may, on certain occasions, determine has been overwhelmed by other considerations or rights. It has been that the right obtains at all only when there
is no overwhelming claim against it. "Alice has a right to genetic privacy" is
true just when the moral reasons for Alice's being entitled to keep information about her genome to herself are more powerful than the reasons for
her to have to disclose; the right is not a further reason, and assertions about
who has what rights over genetic information are the *outcome* of discussions,
not an input to them. In fact, it is not at all obvious what talking about
"rights to privacy" would add to any conversation about who may do what
with whose information when those rights are taken as *data*. It is always open
to us to ask about what it is in virtue of which a person would be able to make
such a claim – which interests are served, or which of another's duties the
putative rights-holder is at liberty to waive.[4]

On the face of it, it looks as though there is likely to be a head-on collision
between the account I have tried to give, and a large tradition (supported by all
kinds of reasons) that thinks about rights in another way. Any such collision is
unlikely to leave my account looking healthy; but it would make barely a dent
on the common-or-garden account of what it is to have a right. For that reason,
for the time being, I want to keep my claim quite minimal. It suffices to say that
adherence to the conventional model of rights *in respect of genetic information
and genetic privacy* gets us into tangles such as that presented by Gerry and
Terry; and the conventional model does not seem to apply all that well to
genetic information. In making this claim, I can leave other aspects of life and
discussion about rights alone. This may be genetic exceptionalism of a kind.
But it may simply be that not every area of moral debate is one in which rights-
talk is applicable, and that problems thrown up by genetics are exemplars of
that point. Neither, in fact, does refusing to treat rights-claims as *data* denude
the remainder of the moral landscape particularly. We can still talk about
people being wronged even when they do not have a relevant right; and we can
still talk about them forgiving the one who wronged them. For example,
Charlie might feel – justifiably – that he was snubbed and thereby wronged
when he was not invited to Dave's party; but it would follow neither that he
must have had a right to be invited, nor that he could not forgive Dave. That
much of the moral language we use can be applied to claims about rights does
not mean that it is always about rights. And for that reason, it is entirely
possible that we are not actually making an exception for genetic information
when we consider moral problems about who should have access to what and
on what terms: for as long as there are other areas where moral terms are
applicable without implying rights or rights-claims, then there will be no exception to be made for genetic information.

And so my claim is not that we ought to ditch rights-talk, or even that we
ought to erase it from the lexicon when we are talking about problems of
access to genetic information: it is the much less ambitious claim that there
likely is not a thoroughgoing *ab initio* right to privacy over genetic information. We can append to this perfectly happily the idea that the language of

privacy rights does nevertheless do service as a useful way of talking about the entitlements that we have come to recognise as being held by a person, or that we would recognise in a person after due moral consideration. We would not say that accessing genetic information about a person is wrong when and because a right is violated, but that we can say a right is violated when and because we think that accessing the information is wrong; and we can say that because the language of rights serves as a useful shorthand way to refer to the outcome of moral deliberation.

Still, there will likely be a nagging doubt that the account I have offered here is undesirable because it is wildly unpredictable. People could only claim as a right whatever claim had turned out to be the most powerful within a given context. Equally, a putative right held against one person at one time may not hold against another person or at another time. This would mean that even if we had reached a conclusion about Alice's entitlement to refuse Bob access to information about her genome in one case, we would not necessarily be any the wiser when it came to others. Neither would her failure to establish that she had anything that we could call a privacy right against Charlie tell us anything much about whether her claims would also fail against Dave.

But a willingness to talk about the entitlements that we would recognise in a person after due moral consideration indicates how some of the worries about unpredictability and instability could be soothed. Nothing in the idea that there is no *ab initio* right to genetic privacy implies that there will not be patterns that fit fairly well in almost all cases: the core criteria for moral judgement would be pretty stable, and so the use of the word "right" in the context of such judgements would be generally uncontroversial. Admittedly, "almost all cases" will leave the possibility that there will be situations in which a pattern cannot be satisfactorily applied. But since there are problematic cases anyway, the overall picture would not really be all that different. Although *ABC v St George's* as adjudicated turned on a question about duties of care, the parties were talking at root about what they held to be conflicting rights: XX's right to privacy *versus* his daughter's right to know about her possible genetic inheritance. Settling the question involved working out whose was the stronger claim. Did the claimant win because she had the stronger right, or is "rights" a shorthand for the reasons why she won? In some senses, it makes no difference. But if we opt for the first interpretation, it is still open to us to wonder *why* her rights were the stronger – and, in making the decision, why her rights *would* be stronger. In other words, so long as we treat a case like *ABC* as being a case in which rights were in conflict, the important questions will not have gone away. Recasting the dispute as a conflict of *claims to rights*, rather than as a conflict of fully-fledged rights, arguably helps to think about the problem more clearly. At the very worst, it removes a layer of grime and thereby helps us get a better view of the moral picture and all its details.

iii. Exceptionalism and Unconfinement, Again

As I indicated in chapter 1, "genetic exceptionalism", whereby questions raised by genetic technologies and information are treated as being qualitatively different from other questions, is largely disparaged within bioethics. All the same, the case against genetic privacy rights as a *datum* of ethical, legal, and regulatory debate has been built upon a characteristic that is, even if not unique to genetic information, then at least not present in respect of most other kinds of information: it is unconfined. Were genetic information confined, the Gerry and Terry problem would evaporate: Gerry could find out about his genome without violating any informational privilege, and hence any putative right to privacy, that Terry might claim; Terry could refuse to share his own genetic information without thereby risking the transformation of something private into something taboo. Equally, on a theoretical level, it is much easier to make sense of rights to privacy as rights to control personal information, or to control access to the self, if we are confining our inquiry to confined information. As such, it looks as though there may be a line to be drawn between genetic information, *qua* unconfined, and other kinds of information; we have to think about them differently. And if we have to think about them differently, then we do seem to find ourselves back in a situation that is perhaps not exactly *exceptionalism* in respect of genetic information, but at least *differentiation*. Yet we ought not to be beguiled by this; it's simply a matter of noting that while there may be more interested parties in respect of genetic information than in respect of other kinds, and while those interests may intersect with each other in unexpected ways, we can still say that the fundamental questions are the same across the board. We will want to know who has what right; and if it turns out that nobody can make a convincing claim to have a right in a given situation, we can still ask meaningfully about the interplay of their interests. *What* we have to think about when we are thinking about who ought to have what kind of access to genetic information and on what terms may be different from what we would think about when we are thinking about who should have access to other kinds of information; but *how* we think about it need not differ at all.

The argument in the second half of chapter 6 attempted to show that there might be normative considerations in favour of putting a putative right to genetic privacy to one side and favouring other people's moral claims even if there were an argument that provided a convincing theoretical explanation of what a right to genetic privacy would be. Whatever we think about the presence or otherwise of a right to privacy in principle, there may be reasons to think that certain others have an interest in aspects of our genetic information in a way that they would not one in respect of other information, and that interest may be substantial. It might be tempting simply to say that we have a conflict of rights in such situations. But is it really the rights that conflict, or the *claims*? If Alice and Bob claim to have a right to the exclusive use of some good φ but we are inclined to think that on balance it should be

Alice who gets it, then it is not obvious what practical difference Bob's right would make. For sure, Bob would still be entitled to have his claim taken seriously; but when it comes down to it, if Alice and Bob have equal and opposite rights to φ, then those rights cancel out. If they have unequal rights, then it is the factor in virtue of which those rights are unequal that counts, rather than their having a right *per se*. Either way, it keeps things more straightforward to bracket the rights-talk, at least until we have determined that it is Alice's claim that we have the greater reason to endorse. But there need be nothing special about genetic information here, and so there is no need to worry about exceptionalism.

On this normative front, questions about who has a legitimate interest in control over information, and so about who has the practical right to control it, may not alter much according to whether we are talking about genetic information: if viewed from a sufficiently narrow perspective, Perry's interest in information that would be relevant to the price of the insurance policy she is setting up for Kerry will not hinge on whether Kerry's risks are genetic. But how narrow a perspective is *proper* may nevertheless be different in respect of confined and unconfined information. If Perry wants to know simply about whether Kerry has been vaccinated against a certain disease, Kerry's relatives Sherry and Cherry would not be implicated; if she wants to know whether Kerry is at risk from a genetic malady, they would. Again, there does seem to be a case to be made for a kind of differentiation, because of the way that genetic information alters the way that we have to balance the competing claims – and to think about who the referent of the information would be. Again, though, this is not really exceptionalism, because the *process* for deciding whose right has the normative heft to make a moral difference need not be fundamentally different according to whether we are talking about genetic or somatic information.

Something else is worth pointing out here. I claimed in chapter 2 that there is something of a tendency to conflate the private and the confidential. I suggested that the private refers to that which is not (or not yet) in the interpersonal realm, and an implication of this is that duties of privacy amount to duties not to bring otherwise-private information into the light; duties of confidentiality have to do with how we should treat information that another person (usually the referent) has brought into the interpersonal realm. If Alice tells Bob something that Charlie has an interest in knowing, we would be looking at questions of whether Bob has a duty of confidentiality and what that would entail; if Bob discovers something about Alice without her telling, then it is privacy that is engaged. But decisions about the proper course of action in respect of both privacy and about confidentiality will all draw on the kinds of principle that I surveyed in the last chapter, and the ways in which those principles interact. In other words, though I began this inquiry asking about genetic *privacy*, the points I have made apply to all contexts in which information is being handled. The fundamental idea – that rights-claims in respect of the control of this information are outcomes rather than *data* of debate – ought to apply just as well in principle to privacy and confidentiality.

iv. Reading Rights

With all this in mind, we have reached an appropriate point to have a quick look at the way the literature has handled some areas in which concerns about genetic privacy are raised. I make no claim that what follows is a systematic survey of the literature: I make no bones about it being a sample of what some people have argued about some topics.

(a) Direct-to-Consumer Genetic Testing

The fall in the price of genetic sequencing has meant that direct-to-consumer (DtC) genetic testing of one sort or another is accessible to almost everyone: a kit that enables us to find out about our own genomes and ancestry is not an unusual Christmas present – a possibility that would have seemed wildly implausible just a generation ago. The availability of such kits raises a range of ethical questions about consent, about preparedness for (and the potential harm of) unexpected and undesirable discoveries, and so on. By and large, though we may sometimes be sceptical about the wisdom of making use of such kits, informed consent for such tests is not a concern in its own right: they are not things that are suggested by others, and so are not things that one has done to one. They are things that one seeks out and does for oneself, non-compulsorily; one does not have to give consent for this sort of thing.[5] Relatedly, Effy Vayena is broadly sanguine about direct-to-consumer tests, seeing them as potentially autonomy-enhancing.[6] Though one may discover things about oneself (or the genetic ingredients of that self, at any rate) from such tests, and though it may be wise sometimes to seek out genetic counselling, one may make surprising discoveries about oneself in any context; there is no particular problem here. Some concern has been raised that ancestry-tracing tests may tell people things that they did not want to know about their ancestry. On the other hand, it is not clear why this really needs to be a big problem. Discovering that you are not related to the people who brought you up, or that you have unknown cousins, need make no deep impact. If you were happy up to this point, it is not obvious why you would be any less so henceforth. Besides, this is not really a privacy problem.

A bigger concern from the perspective privacy is that DtC genetic testing tells us things about others, and that it may mean that information about ourselves is accessible by third parties. Kyle van Oosterum has articulated two aspects to this concern: first, that one's genetic information may (and will) be accessed by others should it be passed on to third parties, which is a diminution of privacy; second, that finding something out about yourself may generate an obligation to report it to third parties: for him, this would undermine autonomy, but it may also amount to an obligation to surrender one's own privacy.[7] On top of this, DtC tests obviously raise versions of the Gerry and Terry problem, insofar as that anyone who makes use of one will also perforce learn about blood relatives, thereby violating their privacy and putative privacy rights.

But does any of this really raise concerns about privacy *rights*? It is not obvious that it would. When it comes to potential obligations to inform third parties, the concerns about autonomy and about privacy both seem small. On the autonomy front, if there is a moral obligation to inform, then there is nothing more to be said: that morality requires that we φ or refrain from ψ is hardly a complaint. I cannot deny my obligation not to murder by pointing out that it constrains my freedom to murder, and the same applies to any other obligation. This speaks to the privacy point, too: if third parties have a sufficiently large interest in accessing the information from a DtC kit consumer's genome, then that user's privacy may be on the line, but his or her *right* to privacy will not be because *ex hypothesi* there would have been no such right. This does, of course, raise its own questions concerning what a sufficient interest is. Oosterum draws our attention to medical research companies, for example. Working out whether they have a sufficient interest in accessing information may well involve thinking about the importance of and warrant for a given piece of research, or even of research broadly conceived. For example, we might think that there is a significant good to be had in knowing about a correlation between certain genes and, say, susceptibility to bowel cancer, and that therefore a violation of privacy stands a tolerable chance of being warranted (especially if the information is anonymised and kept under tight control); but digging into genetic databanks in the hope of learning about the genetic basis for our preferences for bitter chocolate or coffee is, on the face of it, trivial: it may not provide a sufficient warrant for accessing the information, irrespective of how well controlled it is. And this is important when it comes to privacy, since maintaining privacy is a matter of leaving things be: to violate privacy is to snuffle things out, and the permissibility of such snuffling will depend on the moral warrant the snuffler has to snuffle.

This does not mean that DtC providers, having built up an archive of information about clients, are entirely at liberty to sell it on, even for the sake of a good cause, unless those clients are aware from the start that such use may be made of the information about them and given the chance to opt out. One important reason for this is that clients have paid for the service. There is something very disquieting about DtC firms taking money from clients who want to learn something about themselves, and then selling on the information revealed. The issue may be one of a breach of confidentiality – much will depend here on the client's awareness that the information may be shared – but it is compounded by a whiff of profiteering. By analogy, if I commission an architect to build me a house and that architect then uses the design for which I paid to build someone else's house, I might think this a little morally shabby, even if there were no exclusivity clause in our contract: after all, I had paid for a service to *me*.[8] Similarly, if I pay the builder for materials, then even if I don't want the leftover bricks and have no problem with his using them elsewhere, his *charging* the second person looks as though he is exploiting a resource that I have provided, and so exploiting me.

But though this is a question about who has access to what, it is not really a concern about privacy.

Naturally, this concern is less powerful if the information is passed on for free. But even here, it seems straightforward enough to say that clients' having provided samples with certain expectations and not others generates *a reason* not to pass on information. That said, not all reasons are conclusive. Just as, so I shall suggest in a moment, criminal justice may sometimes generate a reason to share information, so might a reasonable hypothesis about how to treat an unpleasant medical condition.

However, since genetic information is unconfined, in signing up for DtC genetic testing one also enlists members of one's family. This may imperil their privacy, because it may mean that information of which they are the secondary referent is brought to the DtC company's attention. Not everyone will be particularly concerned by this: for someone whose position regarding privacy and privacy rights is broadly consonant with an Access to Self account, the thought might be that so long as the information is anonymised, nobody will be able to complain that their self or extended self has been accessed. Whether it is possible to guarantee that it would remain anonymised in an age of big data is a further question; but even here, deanonymisation would require an effort by the de-anonymising agent, and it is likely that that in itself would be sufficient to raise concerns about a violation of the principle of humility – the principle of knowing when not to impose oneself on the world. Merely seeking out information that one has no particular reason, or no defensible reason, to seek out would be sufficient to establish wrongfulness.

What about lingering worries that Lenny's having agreed to contribute to a genetic database has *de facto* enlisted Benny, Jenny, Kenny, and Penny into that same database, potentially without their knowledge and consent? This is a concern that I am willing to face down. If the argument presented here is correct, then none of Lenny's siblings or parents has an *ab initio* right to genetic privacy, and therefore there is no right violated from the bare fact that their "joint stock" genome has been shared (and certainly not if the information is anonymous). Neither is it obvious that there would be any particular reason to think that Lenny had acted in a particularly blameworthy way, at least so long as he had been minimally solicitous of his family's likely desires, and so there would be correspondingly little reason to suppose that his family had an enormous cause for complaint – at least, provided that he was not profiting from it in a way that prevented them from doing likewise. But it is not easy to imagine any such situation in which that might be an issue.

(b) Third-Party Access

My argument over the past few paragraphs, and in chapter 6, has set the scene for claims about third-party access to genetic information, and so there is probably little that I need to add. An insurer may have a claim to access genetic information; whether that claim is sufficiently powerful to generate an entitlement to do so will depend on the circumstances. Would using the information be actuarially fair? If it were, would actuarial fairness correlate to justice *senso latu*? That is, would actuarial fairness make a difference to the accessibility of basic goods? The greater the adverse effect on the person whose genome is in question, the more concerned we are likely to be about the use of information about that genome – and since there is no point in having access to the information if not to use it, the more concerned we would have reason to be about that access. Beyond a certain point, we would be able to say that access would not be justified; and that would suffice to generate a right in the referent not to have that information accessed – which is another way of saying that it would, *beyond this point* (the identification of which would be the task of public deliberation) generate a right to privacy.

A slightly trickier problem is posed by police access to genetic information. It is obvious that law-enforcement agencies' ability to use DNA evidence in identifying and prosecuting perpetrators can be very desirable. There is any number of rapists, murderers, and the like who have been brought to justice on the basis of DNA evidence. I take it that nobody would want to deny that this is a good thing. That having been allowed, though, it is apparently only a small step to saying that the police ought to have access to DNA databases in order to seek out matches, and thereby to close in on suspects. I have already mentioned the so-called Golden State Killer, who was tracked down by just such means. And when the crime in question is particularly heinous, there may well be good reason to suppose that there is sufficient reason for the information to be made available, albeit perhaps with safeguards, such as it being the databank owner who checks a sample provided by the police, rather than the police being given a free pass to the databank.

That it does seem to matter who carries out the evidential search speaks to a qualm that we might have with the next obvious step: granted that genetic sequencing is so cheap, and is likely to get cheaper, and granted that it is desirable to catch perpetrators of heinous crimes so that they can be punished or rehabilitated or simply kept away from the public, why not build up a population-wide databank for forensic purposes? We could imagine existing databanks being combined and made available, and a blood test being taken from every neonate or newly-registered citizen, to aid with the speedy solution of crimes. And if we've nothing to hide from such a system, then we have nothing to fear, do we?

This last sentence is the key to what is troubling about unlimited police access to genetic data. Even assuming that the criminal laws on the statute book are unimpeachably just, then there *is* something to fear from such a system. And what there is to fear is a fundamental shift in the familiar model of the relationship between the individual and the state – a shift from a world in which everyone is assumed to be innocent until proven otherwise and the onus is on the state to identify and provide a rationale for the identification of suspects, to a world in which everyone is assumed to be if not exactly guilty, still at least not exactly innocent, and the onus shifts, however slightly, to the accused.[9]

So it may well be that something like the principle of solidarity for the woman attacked would give men a good reason to provide a sample for sequencing in the aftermath of a rape; and it might be that one of those donations is from a close relative of the perpetrator. In such cases, it would seem like a stretch for the perpetrator to complain that his privacy had been violated. (On this at least, Kaye seems to be right when he points out that "not all aspects of the freedom to be left alone, or even the freedom to be left alone from governmental demands for bodily specimens are equally momentous".[10]) There may also be good reasons not to worry too much about the complaints of the person who provided the sample about his control over his genetic information being diminished: partly this is because we might think that the public good in prosecuting perpetrators is sufficient, but also partly because approaching him for consent may generate a small but nontrivial risk that he would tip off the suspect, and his all-things-considered small loss of control is therefore warranted. However, the solidarity that led someone to provide a sample cannot be mandated, and so for the police to keep those DNA profiles on file for future reference would be more likely to be unacceptable, and its permissibility would have to be argued for on its own terms: again, it would be bringing information into, or keeping information in, the interpersonal or public realm when there is no specific need. "To provide a resource in the event of future crime" is *a* reason to keep hold of the information; but (especially granted the low probability that any single donor to the databank will be a perpetrator,[11] and the low probability that knowing that one's DNA is stored is any kind of deterrent[12]) it is plausible to think that it pales into insignificance when compared to the pernicious shift in the relationship between police and public. On these grounds, even if a universal genetic databank were to be preferable to police using DtC data for the sake of privacy protections, there would be other public policy reasons to resist such a move. DtC companies' databanks represent a resource that it may be good to use; that goodness is not in itself a warrant for creating other databanks.

And not all criminal laws are unimpeachable anyway. Rape is the sort of thing that ought to be illegal; but there could be other things that a wicked regime would make illegal that are perfectly morally permissible, and we would not want to endorse as acceptable sweeps of the genetic databases if that would serve repression. That said, if a government is determined to pass morally suspect legislation, complaining about the permissibility of accessing genetic information in their enforcement is perhaps a secondary concern. When talking about what governments should and should not be doing, we must assume that they are at least prepared to pretend to be morally constrained.

(c) Duties to Warn

Though the case of *ABC v St George's* ostensibly hinged in practice over duties of care, one does not have to scratch the surface too deeply to see that the fundamental question under consideration was one of the duties of a healthcare professional to tell a patient's relatives that they may be carrying a gene associated with a particular medical condition – in this case, Huntington's. Many people have argued that the carrier of certain genes may have a duty to inform relatives; but this leaves open the question of what ought to be done when they refuse.

The argument that I have been building would mean that framing matters such as this in terms of whether the right to be told about one's (possible) genetic inheritance is more important than the right to confidentiality is to make the question more difficult to answer than it need be. If we think that there is an *ab initio* right held by either party in a dispute like this, then there is no obvious and non-dogmatic reason to deny the inverse right to the other. If those rights are equal and opposite, then they will cancel out and leave us having to decide who should have what sort of access to or control over the information in question either by weighing up moral reasons other than rights, or by adverting to some non-moral mechanism. Even if they are not equal and opposite, we might still wonder in virtue of what it is that one of those claimed rights comes out as more powerful than the other.

Instead, we should be thinking about the principles that would inform the actions of all interested parties, and the potential consequences of each option. A relevant professional will have a moral reason to warn relatives and a moral reason not to, the first perhaps based in something like a principle of beneficence, and the second perhaps based in something like a principle of fidelity – although this will not exhaust the possibilities, and it will not tell us about the limits of those principles.[13] Decisions about how to act in cases like this may be informed by analogies with other information. For example, a healthcare professional who has been told something supposedly in confidence about something reprehensible that the patient has done will have to decide whether her behaviour in respect of that information can be bounded by the principle of fidelity: there will be some things that the principle would not cover. Similarly, informing public health authorities about the notifiable disease diagnosis of a patient who made it clear that he will not inform them himself may be a breach of confidence; but whether it is permissible will be a further matter: it may be. Moreover, decisions like these may be informed by whether they relate to keeping a confidence, or keeping a secret: we may weigh these things differently. Bringing things back to genetics, informing a person that a close blood relative is a carrier of a particular gene may be a breach of confidence. But it also seems likely that not informing would, in some cases, tip over from maintaining the primary referent's confidentiality to keeping a secret from the relative. Again, whether or not this makes a normative difference, it certainly does make a difference to the *kind* of problem that must be solved.

I suggested in chapter 2 that one does not need to be taken into anyone's confidence to learn something secret about them, and so there may be no confidentiality to breach (and no principle of fidelity engaged). This may mitigate the putative wrong of telling, especially if we are inclined to think that confidentiality is an aspiration but that keeping secrets would be morally fishy. Or it may be that telling would require going behind the patient's back, which would make things worse. These are the sorts of things that we might expect to find playing on the mind of Emma, the geneticist from chapter 3, when she is considering whether to tell Terry about the potentially worrying results of Gerry's genetic test. Much will depend on things like penetrance, the likelihood of morbidity, and so on; there is no reason to suppose that an answer would be both neat and generalisable. But for this reason alone, we have cause to think that trying to persuade the primary referent to tell would not always be enough.[14]

A fascinating take on the putative duties to warn about genetic timebombs arises from the suggestion that there may be times when there is a duty to self-censor. Taking a lead from Anita Allen, Earl Spurgin suggests a couple of situations in which morality seems to require that we *not* share information, even about ourselves. One of these is the standard too-much-information scenario: it is safe to presume that we ought to hold back from talking about sexual or defecatory matters in graphic detail over Christmas dinner, and we would not make the problem go away if we tried to reassure our listeners that we really didn't mind sharing these details with them. But the other argument is that we may have a duty to self-censor when not to do so would impose undue burdens on others. Trivial examples of this are easy to give: we ought not to speak when we are in the theatre. But Spurgin has in mind something a bit more radical, mooting the possibility that (for example) teachers might have a duty not to complain about their students online, because even if nobody is wronged or acts wrongly in such cases, "their superiors must use valuable time to defend them against the charges of customers, students, parents, guardians, and others who become enraged after reading their posts".[15] This creates an unreasonable burden for those superiors, and therefore such complaints ought to be restrained. Presumably, we could extend the argument, and wonder whether a person who has been given the results of a genetic test might sometimes have a duty to keep quiet if he thinks that that would place a burden on blood relatives.

Some of the details of this take do not seem to me to be plausible, amounting to the claim that Alice ought not to make certain perfectly defensible statements in public for fear that Bob might misunderstand them and Charlie might make a point of imputing malice, thereby compelling Diane to waste time talking Bob and Charlie down. This makes all speakers ultimately responsible for the misapprehensions of their listeners. However, the appeal to unreasonable burdens is suggestive all the same. It may be that my knowing about my own genome and sharing that information with others creates burdens. As Allen herself has admitted in considering possible reasons to self-censor, "[m]y genome is also my siblings' genome, so I have an obligation to protect the privacy of my genome".[16] Anyone who has been persuaded by my arguments in this book will want to resist the head-first insistence that there is an obligation to protect the privacy of my own genome; but this is compatible with thinking that there are reasons to resist informational profligacy. Telling third parties about myself is also telling them about my siblings; though I may be unashamed by some fact about my genome, and though I may think that they ought to be unashamed as well, the point would stand that they may *not* be. And there may be reasons other than shame in play, too: even if we think that they really ought to inform their insurer about a particular genetic risk, it does not follow that we may do the job for them. To be clear: it is possible that we may tell. But we have to make the case, not simply assume it.

v. Legal Rights and the Challenge of Specificationism

Allowing that my account of the ethics of genetic privacy rights is correct, or at least tolerably close to being correct, what are its implications for law? It looks at first glance like there may be difficulties. It is one thing to embrace uncertainty and say that moral claims may be subject to dispute in the way they get manifested in real cases; but we expect law to be much more stable and predictable. It is reasonable to think that a good law would be one that tracks the contours of morality; but if we hold to that doctrine here, it looks as though we'd be committed to the idea that a good law would be beyond our reach, because it would have to be incredibly finely-grained in its drafting to be able to capture the details and nuances of the relationship between all parties in all situations. Such a law would be all-but-impossible to draft and to apply. The concern is that we may have opened the door to a kind of specificationism.

A specificationist account of rights – and "specificationist" is a word that tends to get used as an objection rather than as a badge (though, to be fair, specificationism as an approach is something that some are willing to endorse[17]) – would hold that whatever rights we hold are highly context-dependent, and so much less pervasive than one might otherwise have thought. What looks like a reasonably straightforward absolute right to φ would, for a specificationist, need a lot more unpacking. Feinberg illustrates the specificationist objection by considering the example of possibly the most intuitive absolute moral and legal right – the right to life:

> A philosopher friendly to the idea of absolute human rights might argue that all simple and brief statements of (say) the right to life are of necessity mere abbreviations for an elaborately complex statement defining a right that is absolute. The fuller statement would begin, presumably, by stating that all "human beings" (a phrase itself in need of detailed definition) have a right not to be killed. It would then proceed to explain what is to be understood by "killing" and which circumstances – described in a general, but not too general, way – constitute exceptions (this could lead to a discussion of war, capital punishment, and

self-defense, among other topics). The statement would include a discussion of what priority rules are to be used for determining who has the right and who does not in situations of unavoidable conflict; again, these rules would be described in a general, but not too general, way. A similarly detailed statement would follow, describing the full extent, within carefully circumscribed limits, of the right to be rescued. Clearly such an enterprise would yield a book-length statement at the very least.[18]

Trying to legislate for every instance in which a right to life may be engaged would be bordering on the fractal, with every stipulation inviting qualifications and subclauses, and each qualification and subclause inviting another. The general concern would translate to any attempt to articulate legal rights to genetic privacy. Presumably, we would need a full account of which genes are in question – their penetrance, the age of the agents (in order to calculate whether a given gene will be likely to have any effect before they die of other causes), which agents count, which interests count, perhaps some biographical details of the agents, and so on. All this done, for the right to have any particular practical salience, the claims of each agent would have to be measured against the claims of all other relevant agents, which would appear to require the formulation of some common standard by which they could be measured. Such a task would be huge: we would be waiting a long time before any clear guidance was produced, and real-life cases would be piling up in the meantime. If this were to be the way that we tried to accommodate the view of rights I have adopted here into law, it would imply that law would be incredibly unstable, or impracticable.

But on reflection, it turns out that worries like this need not concern us too much. For one thing, we might want simply to bulldoze our way through the concern, reminding ourselves that what law can do and morality cannot is make stipulations. Lawmakers get to make rules as they see fit. Tracking morality as closely as possible may be desirable, but law is not simply codified morality, and morality is not the only consideration in lawmaking: efficiency and utility are also important. More, while there may be justifiable complaint if and to the extent that law fails to protect things that we hold to be moral rights, there would be no corresponding complaint if law gives rights that do not have a strong moral foundation. And so if lawmakers decide that there are policy reasons to posit a thoroughgoing legal right to genetic privacy, then a thoroughgoing legal right to genetic privacy there will be, even if that ignores some of the nuances of moral debate. These lawmakers would presumably be creating legal rights that they hope will capture the balance of moral considerations in most cases, and leaving it at that. Perhaps nobody will get quite the legal rights that they wanted, but in that, the situation would not be significantly different from any other area of law. The legal right would still aspire to reflect the moral situation; and that is probably all that we could legitimately expect. As such, it may be possible to imagine, and to endorse, a legal system that simply stipulates that privacy rights when it comes to genetic information are *thus* and *so*.

On the other hand, the naïve introduction of legal rights may store up problems should they lead to self-evident moral problems. For example: imagine that a law was passed stipulating that nobody may access genetic information about another without that other's written consent. It may be that such a law enjoyed a great deal of public support – but it would, very quickly, generate myriad problems simply because genetic information is unconfined, and the law would generate a whole nation of Gerrys and Terrys. Any reasonably plausible law would either have to be highly specific, or else have built into it a great deal of room for interpretation. (In this light, it is notable that Article 8 rights under the European Convention, which would most closely relate to problems about access to and control over genetic information, are rights to *respect for* private and family life – not respect for privacy; what "respect for" entails is a further question, and it is right that it is left un-prescribed.) Some kind of evaluation of the relevant interests will be a necessary part of applying the law: it turns out that evaluative aspects cannot be separated from the practice of any legal system that is plausibly supple and usable.

But it ought to be possible to steer a course between the twin vices of a blithe positivism that is indifferent to detail, and an absurd specificationism that is mired in it. It is reasonable to expect that, notwithstanding the possible permutations of the moral picture I outlined in the last chapter, there will be broad patterns of morally permissible and impermissible access to genetic information from which it ought to be possible to derive at least a framework for legislation. Hard cases that do not fit easily into the established pattern, and that are unforeseen by the drafters of law, may crop up from time to time. But this is not a particular problem – no more than would beset any other piece of legislation – because law can, and must, deal with complexity without codifying every conceivable turn of events. So it is that something like the tort of negligence is part of law without there being a precise prescribed standard for behaviour fine-tuned to every context; the law here revolves around the reasonability of decisions that people might make in the circumstances. (Even the criminal law can have something of this flexibility: granted a law that outlaws homicide, questions about the proper response to it are perfectly capable of being shaped around considerations such as whether the killing was premeditated, a mercy-killing, motivated by personal gain, and so on. All these will feed into whether we think of the homicide as murder or something else, and what kind of punishment we would think appropriate. Context matters even here.)

There is no reason at all to suppose that an attempt to legislate for rights to genetic privacy, and to apply any such law, would not follow this sort of model, with legal as well as moral entitlements in hard cases decided according to what is reasonable given the circumstances, and with precedents helping shape the rough-hewn ends of statute.[19] In most cases, the rules determining who is entitled to access to what information will be easy to deduce and apply; but as with something like negligence, even when they are not, there would still be scope for an appropriately qualified panel to determine propriety. This is because, even for the novel case, there will be patterns of inference that can be drawn from the past and applied in the present. Decisionmaking in this sense – moral and legal – would be a matter of deciding whether terms like "privacy right" would be properly applicable, and properly judged to be held by whom, in a given situation. As in the moral case, an agent would have a right to genetic privacy just in those circumstances in which their claim to control the flow of information was more powerful than the claim of others to access it.

vi. Professional Guidance

The relationship between law and professional guidance is not a one-way street. Obviously, it will not be possible for professional codes to allow or require what the law forbids, though they may forbid or require things that the law allows. But professional standards and guidelines can in themselves influence the law, and the way that the law is applied. Most obviously, the test for the tort of negligence is sometimes provided by an assessment of whether an agent has breached the standards of behaviour deemed appropriate in this or that context, with professional guidance documents helping to formulate that propriety test. More generally, a legislature might delegate the formation of certain norms that will be legally enforceable to professional bodies. In this way, professional standards are constrained by law, and law is informed by professional standards. Further, just as lawmakers can posit rules about what one ought to do irrespective of whatever moral complexities there may be, so the same applies to professional bodies: it is within their gift to be quite prescriptive. Yet law has a reason to allow for the exercise of judgement and has the resources to do so, and the same applies to the professions and their guidance.

As it happens, the moral picture that I have been painting – in which rights are not *data* of moral decisionmaking but things we ascribe at the end of a process of decisionmaking and as a way of crystallising and articulating the decisions made – is already reasonably close to what we see in practice. When it comes to things like privacy, the extant guidelines that direct medical practice call on practitioners to make judgements about whether a breach is warranted in this or that context. For example, the legal annex of the latest version of the GMC's ethics guidance on information disclosure states that

> It is generally accepted that the common law allows disclosure of confidential information if:
>
> a   the patient consents
> b   it is required by law, or in response to a court order
> c   it is justified in the public interest.[20]

There are quibbles that we might raise here: there is a risk of conflation of privacy and confidentiality, and it is a little unhelpful for a statement to say that the law allows disclosure of confidential information if it is required by law. Still, we can see that there is a great deal of room here for interpretation. Assuming that "justified" here is taken not in the "thin" or legalistic sense of "capable of being presented as a reason for action" but in the more robust (though potentially question-begging) sense of "being shown to be the proper reason for action", then it will fall to practitioners and those with whom they may choose to confer and consult to make a call on whose claim concerning the control of information is the stronger, and this decision will draw on a decision about what counts as the public interest to begin with.

There is similar room for interpretation under the GMC's rehearsal of other sources of law. In explaining the requirements of the General Data Protection Regulation, it notes that disclosure of health information may be permissible if it is "necessary to protect the vital interests of the data subject or another person in a case where the data subject is physically or legally incapable of giving consent" or if "the processing is necessary for reasons of substantial public interest".[21] And in respect of the Human Rights Act, it notes that

> Any interference with a person's right to privacy must be a necessary and proportionate response to the situation. This means there must be a fair balancing of competing interests. These include:
>
> - the potential damage caused to the individual whose privacy will be breached
> - society's interest in the provision of a confidential health service
> - the public interest that will be achieved through breaching the individual's privacy.[22]

Clearly, in all these statements, a great deal is left to interpretation. What is the public interest, and what does "substantial" mean? How is that public interest to be measured against other considerations? When we are making assessments of proportionality, what is the standard – and how do we decide what a fair balancing of interests would mean? There is no clear rule that one may do *this* but not *that*. Rather, the permissibility or otherwise of an action is a matter of judgement; proper judgement will be determined by whether criteria of fairness and proportionality are properly applied. This point brings us back to the position I outlined in the last chapter: determining whether something is fair or proportional will require nothing more than the analysis of whether words such as "fair" and "proportional" would be applicable to it, or whether they would better fit some modified course of action. In cases like this, argumentation from analogy would be invaluable. In turn, all this is an indication that, insofar as that this guidance tells us anything useful about rights to privacy at all – and notwithstanding that a right to privacy is taken as a baseline – it does so only if those rights are outputs from, rather than inputs to, a system of deliberation. Correspondingly, when the statement talks about a person's right to privacy, and based on the argument I have been making, we ought to tread carefully, and treat the word "right" with some care – perhaps mentally substituting in the phrase "claimed right".

Neither is this state of affairs limited to the United Kingdom. The American Medical Association's guidance on privacy includes as Opinion 3.1.1 the statement that

> Physicians must seek to protect patient privacy in all settings to the greatest extent possible and should:
>
> a   Minimize intrusion on privacy when the patient's privacy must be balanced against other factors.
> b   Inform the patient when there has been a significant infringement on privacy of which the patient would otherwise not be aware.
> c   Be mindful that individual patients may have special concerns about privacy in any or all of these areas.[23]

That privacy should be protected "to the greatest extent possible" does not seem to be the language of privacy rights as *data*. And this is because, as I indicated in the chapters up to this point, it is not usual to think that rights ought to be balanced against other factors, on pain of their devolving to "mere" reasons for action. Equally, the call for balance is doing the same work as the GMC's calls for fairness and proportionality; but there is no prescription about what striking it may look like. Context will be crucial. Treating the guidance as articulating a reason for action, which we may subsequently translate into the language of rights should we be so inclined, seems to be the most parsimonious way to interpret guidelines such as this.

vii. Privacy Rights, Reconstructed

So my proposal that a right to privacy ought not to be seen as a *datum* to be weighed against other *data*, but as something that may or may not be assigned based on an assessment of a range of competing claims and considerations, fits in reasonably well with real-world guidance. That assessment will be – at root – a matter of deciding whether words like "proportionate" and "fair" are properly applied in the context. When a practitioner, or anyone else, is asked to act in a way that is proportionate and fair, what is being asked is that a survey of the relevant interests and principles be conducted, and an account offered of which is the most pressing in the context; if a disinterested and moderately competent user of the language would describe this account as capturing the demands of fairness and proportionality, then that is all the evidence that there could possibly be that the account *is* proportionate and fair.

All this – ultimately, the decision about who has what entitlements in respect of genetic information in a given situation – will be informed by precedent decisions and by, fundamentally, linguistic aptitude: of having a sense of which words to use and when, in the light of all the morally-relevant considerations (or as many as a human mind can handle). If there is some irreducible ambiguity, this simply means that there is equipoise: it ought not to make a moral – or legal – difference which route is chosen. Conversely, a sense that doing one thing rather than another would be morally question-able would serve as an indication that time could and should be spent trying to come up with something that raises fewer quibbles.

But, at least when it comes to genetic information, we ought not to take privacy rights as things that will help us decide that route.

Notes

1 The earliest example of this of which I am aware is Fuller, L, "The Case of the Speluncean Explorers", *Harvard Law Review* 62[4] (1949), *passim*.
2 cf Feinberg, J, *Rights, Justice, and the Bounds of Liberty: Essays in Social Philosophy* (Princeton, NJ: Princeton UP, 1980), p 230.
3 *R v Dudley and Stephens* [1884] 14 QBD 273 DC.
4 I do not intend to wade deeply into the interest-v-choice debate about the nature of rights. If rights reflect interests, then working out who has what rights will mean working out their interests; and working out which rights prevail in cases when they (apparently) clash will mean working out whose interests are the most powerful. Once we had worked out whose rights prevail, we would know what we ought to do, and who was entitled to what. So far so good. But suppose we decide that Alice's interests in φ trump Bob's in ψ. Bob still has those interests, and so presumably he still has the right, albeit in some – slightly perplexing – latent form. But what would that right amount to, beyond being another way to talk about Bob's interest? It is tempting to say that Bob's latent right would help explain why Alice ought to regret doing what Bob would prefer she not do. But why should it be that it is only Bob's having a *right* that would explain that? Alice might have all kinds of other reason to regret having overruled Bob's interests: it still makes perfect sense to say that he has persisting interests that were set back, and that decency, or solidarity, or something like that would require feeling bad about that, without having to take any claim about his rights as givens.

What if rights reflect choices? Here, we would be saying that there is some moral consideration in respect of which Bob ought to defer to Alice's wishes or preferences, and that Alice has a right insofar as that she is able to release Bob from that obligation. But obviously whatever reasons Alice has to release Bob from his obligations cannot be matters of his right: one cannot have a right to be released from obligations on pain of their not being obligations to begin with – and certainly not if that right resides in Bob's being able to relieve Alice of what would have to be her obligation to relieve Bob of his obligation. It is straight-forward enough to say that Alice and Bob both might be making claims about the other's duty, from which they may or may not release them; but, again, it is not clear how the situation is clarified by describing these claims as *rights* so much as interests. Note that a choice theorist need not deny that agents have interests that are morally important: it is simply that interests are not sufficient to demonstrate rights. But describing these claims in terms of rights seems to make the actual moral problem less tractable unless we can, once again, provide an account of what it is by virtue of which Alice's claims against Bob (and her ability to release him from his obligations) trump Bob's claims against Alice (and his ability to release her from hers).

5 There is perhaps a concern about one person obtaining a biosample from another, and using it to obtain genomic information without that other's authorisation; but this is a fairly straightforward case of identity fraud, throwing up no especial problems.

6 Vayena, E, "Direct-to-Consumer Genomics on the Scales of Autonomy", *Journal of Medical Ethics* 41[4] (2014), *passim*.

7 Oosterum, K van, "Privacy, Autonomy and Direct-to-Consumer Genetic Testing: A Response to Vayena", *Journal of Medical Ethics* (2022), doi.org/10.1136/medethics-2021-107999.

8 The law, at least in England, would appear to have no time for my complaint, presuming that (in the absence of any explicit assertion to the contrary) rights over the use of a design remain with the architect: see Adrian, A, "Architecture and Copyright: A Quick Survey of the Law", *Journal of Intellectual Property Law & Practice* 3[8] (2008), pp 524–529 for a quick primer.

9 Oddly, Kaye, and Smith appear to take this as an argument *in favour of* universal coverage: see Kaye, D, & Smith, M, "DNA Identification Databases: Legality, Legitimacy, and the Case for Population-Wide Coverage", *Wisconsin Law Review* 2003[3] (2003), *passim*.

10 Kaye, 2001, p 205.

11 That is to say: even if all violent crime were committed by members of a given demographic group, it would not follow that all members of that demographic group, or even many of them, are perpetrators. It is a perfectly good response to the defence that not all men are a danger to women to point out that *enough* men are dangerous to give women a reason to worry; and yet it is also true that those worries in any given situation may not be warranted. The "Not All Men" slogan may often be deployed in a trite and tin-eared way, but it is not without value; and that value applies, *mutatis mutandis*, to everyone.

12 Krimsky, S, & Simoncelli, T, *Genetic Justice: DNA Databanks, Criminal Investigations, and Civil Liberties* (New York: Columbia UP, 2012), p 145ff.

13 cf Lucassen, A, & Parker, M, "Confidentiality and Serious Harm in Genetics – Preserving the Confidentiality of one Patient and Preventing Harm to Relatives", *European Journal of Human Genetics* 12 (2004), *passim*.

14 cf Knoppers, B, "Genetic Information and the Family: Are We our Brother's Keeper?" *Trends in Biotechnology* 20[2] (2002), p 86; see also Foster, C *et al*, "Testing the Limits of the 'Joint Account' Model
of Genetic Information: A Legal Thought Experiment", *Journal of Medical Ethics* 41[5] (2014), pp 380 & 382

15 Spurgin, E, "Why the Duty to Self-Censor Requires Social-Media Users to Maintain Their Own Privacy", *Res Publica* 25[1] (2019), p 15.

16 Allen, A, "An Ethical Duty to Protect One's Own Information Privacy", *Alabama Law Review* 64[4] (2013), p 852.

17 See, for example, Shafer-Landau, R, "Specifying Absolute Rights", *Arizona Law Review* 37[1] (1995), pp 209–226; Webber, G *et al*, *Leglislated Rights: Securing Human Rights through Legislation* (Cambridge, Cambridge UP, 2018), esp §2.5.

18 Feinberg, *op cit*, pp 227–228.

19 In this light, Foster *et al* (2014) suggest a way in which the Common Law has the resources at its disposal to deal with problems of access to genetic information under the terms of the ECHR.

20 https://www.gmc-uk.org/ethical-guidance/ethical-guidance-for-doctors/
    confidentiality/legal-annex
21 https://www.gmc-uk.org/ethical-guidance/ethical-guidance-for-doctors/
    confidentiality/legal-annex
22 https://www.gmc-uk.org/ethical-guidance/ethical-guidance-for-doctors/
    confidentiality/legal-annex
23 https://www.ama-assn.org/delivering-care/ethics/privacy-health-care

Index

Printed in the United States
by Baker & Taylor Publisher Services